From Priory Cottage to Park Campus

The Story of Occupational Therapy Education in Northampton

Jane Evans

Best Wishes, Anne,
Jane Evans

University of Northampton

Published in 2007 by
The University of Northampton
Park Campus
Boughton Green Road
Northampton
NN2 7AL

ISBN 978-1-906398-00-2

Text copyright © University of Northampton

The right of Jane Evans to be identified as the author
of this work has been asserted by her in accordance with the
Copyright Designs and Patents Act 1988

All rights reserved. No part of this publication may be reproduced,
stored in a retrieval system or transmitted in any form or by any means,
electronic, mechanical, photocopying, recording or otherwise,
without the prior permission in writing of the publisher.

Printed by Stanley L. Hunt (Printers) Ltd, Midland Road,
Rushden, Northamptonshire NN10 9UA

CONTENTS

List of illustrations
Acknowledgements
Foreword
Timeline on the development of occupational therapy

Preface   by Professor Annie Turner

Chapter 1   Beginnings
    History of Occupational Therapy - Founding
        of St. Andrew's School   1

Chapter 2 - Foundations
    Joyce Hombersley 1944 – 1957   15

Chapter 3 - Work, Rest and Play
    Social side of the School under Joyce Hombersley   29

Chapter 4 - Signs of Change
    Elin Dallas 1957 – 1972 (up to inspection of 1966)   48

Chapter 5 - The Watershed
    Changes to the School after 1966 under Elin Dallas   62

Chapter 6 - A Step too far?
    Maria Van Garderen 1972 – 1981   77

Chapter 7 - "To wither on the vine"
    Elizabeth Cracknell 1981 – 1995   97

Chapter 8 – Moving on
    Annie Turner 1995 – 2005   117

Chapter 9 – Looking forward
    Sue Griffiths and Annie Turner 2005 –   130

Conclusion   142

Bibliography

Appendix

List of Illustrations

Unless otherwise stated, the owners of the photographs are St.Andrew's Hospital or the University of Northampton

1. Advertisement for the School, 1948	3
2. Dr. Tennent	7
3. The School building, 1950	9
4. Violet Parry and some of the students, 1951	11
5. Joyce Hombersley (British Jnl of OT)	17
6. Timetable for the 1940s	19
7. Light metal workshop, ca. 1950	21
8. Prelims over! ca. 1950 (Bridget Wyatt)	23
9. Toy making, 1950s	25
10. Weaving with Joyce Hombersley (in the background),1947	26
11. Poem from the 1940s by Anne Dickens (Ridgeway)	28
12. Rheinfelden student hostel, 1949 (unknown source)	31
13. Woodwork, ca. 1950s	33
14. Repairing bicycles, 1950s (Bridget Wyatt)	35
15. Hockey team, 1952 (Bridget Wyatt)	39
16. Sports Day, ca. 1950s (Bridget Wyatt)	44
17. Elin Dallas	51
18. Embroidery class with Miss Dallas (sitting, in black), 1958 (unknown source)	53
19. The Can-Can, 1972	56
20. Priory Cottage, 1997	59
21. Dance class, ca. 1960	64
22. Lowood student hostel, 1960s (unknown source)	67
23. Manfield Orthopaedic Hospital OT Department, 1950s	71
24. Creaton TB Sanatorium, in the garden (Bridget Wyatt)	73
25. 3 Directors of Training, ca. 1990: E.Dallas, E.Cracknell, M.Van Garderen	78
26. Neville Parsons Jones ('PJ')	82
27. St.Nicholas & St.Martin's Orthopaedic Hospital, Pyrford: Occupational therapy for a child	87
28. Basket making	89
29. St.Andrew's Hospital Chapel	93
30. Elizabeth Cracknell, 1984 (E. Cracknell)	101
31. Learning to use an adapted tool to peel a potato, 1984	103
32. Learning to garden	107
33. St. Andrew's Hospital main building	111
34. Moving out of Priory Cottage, 1997 (Chronicle & Echo)	119

35. The Princess Royal opens the Kelmarsh building at
　　　　　　　　　　　　　Park Campus　　　　123
36. The avenue in St. Andrew's Hospital grounds　　127
37. The Kelmarsh building　　　　　　　　　　　133
38. Learning silk screen painting, 2007　　　　　　136
39. Sue Griffiths and Annie Turner, 2007　　　　　139

Acknowledgements

I gratefully acknowledge the help given me by staff and students, both past and present. I know there were many more I could have interviewed, and apologise that time constraints prevented me from doing so; also that we did not have enough room to include more of the photographs that were so kindly sent in. Without the reminiscences, photographs and insights of the staff and students, this book could not have been written. I must also express my thanks to Liz Ridley, the Archivist at St. Andrew's Hospital, and to Beryl Warren who has collected so many interesting items, photographs and papers gathered by the Friends of the School. Ann Wilcock's history of the profession was invaluable to me in helping me set the book in context. Finally, many thanks to St. Andrew's Hospital without whose generous support this book would not have been possible.

Jane Evans

Foreword

The idea of writing the history of occupational therapy education in Northampton emerged as the St Andrew's School of Occupational Therapy moved from the hospital site to its new home within the School of Health Science on Park Campus, Nene College in 1997. The Friends' association which was formed at that time began to collect memories from past students, and as the organisation developed over the next few years, writing the history of occupational therapy education in Northampton became one of its prime objectives.

Having trained at the school myself in the mid 1950s, I am aware that throughout my professional life it has held a central place in my affection and I have grown to realise what a special place it was and still is! It is unique in the history of occupational therapy education in England in that it was the only programme established in a large psychiatric hospital and thus had a quite different origin and background to any other occupational therapy school. This in itself makes the recording of its development worthwhile.

Now, due to the generosity of St. Andrew's Hospital and the Division of Occupational Therapy at the University of Northampton, we have been able to realise this objective and the dream has become a reality. We were very fortunate to commission Jane Evans, a Northampton social historian and librarian, to research and write the history. Her work has been thorough and painstaking, tracing the school from its small beginnings when it was founded by Dr. Thomas Tennent during the Second World War, to its present position as the Division of Occupational Therapy within the School of Health at the University of Northampton. The journey takes us through the decades from the first students recruited at the local Art School in 1941 and shows the developments from formal learning by rote and meticulous craftsmanship, to the identity crisis and period of self-doubt for occupational therapy in the 1970s, the problems of funding and bursaries, the move to Park Campus, and finally the present ethos of research and the philosophical drive of 'Occupation for Health'. Alongside this, Jane traces the development of the profession as well as the changing social and political climates which underpin the development of the occupational therapy profession.

We are pleased that this history will enhance the archives of the profession and add to the knowledge base that will underpin some of its future development. I have been delighted to have been able to be part of the team that supervised the development and launch of this history and would like to thank both St. Andrew's Hospital and the former Friends' association (now embedded in the University Alumni Association) for facilitating its creation.

Beryl Warren
July 2007

Secretary, Friends of OT Education in Northampton 1997 - 2007
Chair of the Council of the College of Occupational Therapists 1986
Head/District OT, Wolfson Medical Rehabilitation Centre 1976 - 1987
Student, St Andrew's School of Occupational Therapy 1953 - 1956

Timeline on the Development of Occupational Therapy as a Profession

taken from A.Turner, M.Foster & S.Johnson, *Occupational Therapy and Physical Dysfunction: Principles, Skills and Practice*, 5th ed. (Edinburgh: Churchill Livingstone, 2002)

End of 19th century An increasing awareness of the value of occupation as a treatment. The term, 'occupational therapy' began to evolve. The emphasis was still very much on the use of occupation within the psychiatric field.

1924 Dr. Elizabeth Casson introduced occupational therapy into her nursing home in Clifton, Bristol, after attending a conference by Professor Sir David Henderson and visiting a newly established occupational therapy school in Philadelphia, USA.

1925 Margaret Fulton, the first qualified occupational therapist to work in the UK (after training in Philadelphia) established an occupational therapy department at the Royal Cornhill Hospital, Aberdeen. Dr. Elizabeth Casson sent Constance Tebbit to train in the USA.

1930 Dr. Casson established the first British occupational training school at Dorset House, with Constance Tebbit as principal.

1932 In Scotland the first professional association was formed. It had 30 members.

1936 The Astley Ainslie school was established in Edinburgh. The Association of Occupational Therapists (A.O.T.) was formed in England.

1938 The first public examinations were held.

1939-1945 The A.O.T. set up short courses for occupational therapy auxiliaries. This could be upgraded to full professional status with further study. The War Emergency Diploma allowed professionals with previous qualifications to qualify as occupational therapists.

1941 St. Andrew's School of Occupational Therapy in Northampton was established as the third English school, London being the second.

1947 The National Health Service Act. Occupational therapy schools were privately funded at this time.

1951 First International Congress run by the A.O.T.

1952 World Federation of Occupational Therapists was inaugurated.

1960/1 The establishment of the Council for the Professions Supplementary to Medicine led to State Registration.

1974 The British Association of Occupational Therapists was formed from a merger between A.O.T. and S.A.O.T.

1977 First European Congress.

1978   The Association divided into: The College of Occupational Therapists (to deal with professional and educational matters) and The British Association of Occupational Therapists (the trade union).
1990s Training to 1st degree level established on all pre-registration courses.

Conversation overheard between two young Irish boys - the second speaker is in a wheelchair

'What's Sheila doing?' – 'She's gone to be an OT.' – 'Oh yea, like Sister Angela.' – 'No, you idiot. Sister Angela is a physio. Sister Bryony is an OT.' – 'What's the difference then?' – 'The difference is, if the physio wants me to exercise, she says, "Paddy Doyle, stick your hand above your head." If the OT wants me to exercise, she says, "Paddy Doyle, be an angel and get me that book down off that shelf up there."'

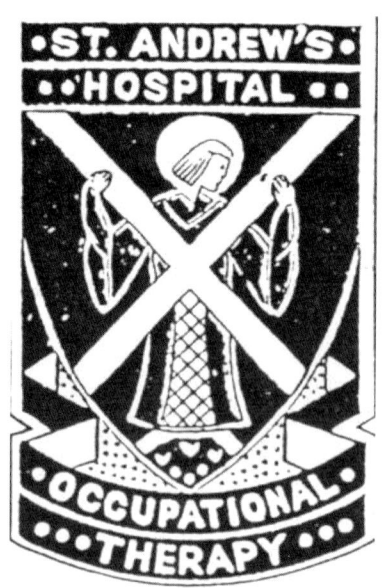

Preface

The concepts behind occupational therapy are not new. Over 2000 years ago Galen, a physician who lived in ancient Greece around 200 AD wrote that *'Employment is nature's best physician and is essential to human happiness'*. However the harnessing of these ideas into the profession of occupational therapy, which believes in the occupational nature of humans and the use of occupation as a means of promoting and maintaining health, is relatively new. The term occupational therapy wasn't in use until the turn of the 20th century, coined by a disabled American architect, George Barton, and the profession only began to establish itself from that time. In 1962 Mary Reilly, an American professor of occupational therapy, captured the essence of the profession's belief in her wonderful statement *'Man, through the use of his hands, as they are energised by his mind and will, can influence the state of his own health'*.

The concepts behind occupational therapy then have had a long gestation but the development of the profession's practice has not always been able to hold fast to these beliefs. At the cusp of the 19th and 20th centuries the practice of occupational therapy clearly reflected the beliefs and cultures of the time. However as it became more established within the health systems in the mid 20th century the profession's philosophy became ontangled and somewhat smothered by the social, political and medical environments in which it was taking root. The portrayal of people's health was dominated by medical thinking based around doctors and diagnoses, while the popularity of the Art and Crafts movement from the beginning of the 20th century was highly influential, focusing occupational therapy's interventions mainly around craft orientated activities. Weaving looms, woodwork and other hand craft prevailed, regardless of the interests of the individual. Work with those who had physical dysfunction used specially developed machinery to exercise particular muscle groups while the ideas of health through doing were cast aside. Therapists working in the field of mental health similarly turned away from the healing power of occupation and developed techniques related to the 'talking therapies'. It wasn't until the 1980s, when occupational therapists began to acquire the graduate skills of research and critical evaluation, that the profession began to question its practice, research and develop its philosophical roots and steer itself back to its philosophical beliefs – a process it continues with today.

It was in the middle of this crucial time that the Northampton School of Occupational Therapy was founded at St Andrew's Hospital in 1941. The school's history therefore is a fascinating reflection of what was happening within the profession and why. This book explores the history of the School from its earliest days to its very changed position in 2007. It charts its development within the social, medical and political climates of the time and reflects how these factors influenced the growth and direction of occupational therapy education in Northampton. The book traces the journeys and experiences of both students and staff and explores some of the political contexts that have shaped, and continue to shape, its development. While the book divides up the history into the periods led by its various principals and professional leaders, it supports the journey with a rich series of anecdotes, mainly from staff and students. It explores therefore, not just the 'what' of happenings but importantly the 'why'.

Here then is a journey of an educational institution that has travelled an important path in the development of a new profession from its early days, through its somewhat unfocused and difficult development, to its present situation of a crystallised philosophy and its growing base of evidence. Clearly the political and social contexts in which professional programmes sit will always shape how occupational therapy education is developed and delivered. But as the profession matures its education offers a range of occupational therapy programmes that enable students to clearly articulate and evaluate what their profession is all about. This enables them to proactively influence its practice and steer it away from, concepts, contexts and practices that constrain and control it towards those that allow it to flourish.

Professor Annie Turner
July 2007

Chapter 1

Beginnings

Original concepts behind occupational therapy – Evidence for the therapy in Ancient Greece, medieval Europe, in England after the Dissolution of the Monasteries and during the Industrial Revolution – Influence on the therapy of the early 20th century Arts and Crafts movement and the physical rehabilitation needs of two World Wars – New freedom for women in early 20th century leading to female careers in care for the sick.

Early 20th century: first course of occupational therapy set up in Boston, USA – 1930 first School set up in Britain – 1933 Government encourages the therapy in mental hospitals - 1941 St. Andrew's Hospital Northampton establishes the third School in England – Course counts as war work – 1943 School recognised officially by the A.O.T. – 1944 Education Act makes students eligible for financial award – 1944 Joyce Hombersley takes over as Principal – Fears that the therapy is becoming too physically orientated.

We have heard that the concepts that underpin occupational therapy are not new. As we have seen, as far back as 200 AD Galen saw that *'Employment is nature's best physician and is essential to human happiness.'* These words explain the essence of occupational therapy. In the 4th century BC Hippocrates, the father of medicine, was prescribing his patients activities such as wrestling, riding and physical labour in the belief that there was a link between the health of the mind and the health of the body. Throughout medieval Europe this philosophy continued, and was followed by the monastic orders, one of whose tasks was to look after the mentally ill. In England after the Dissolution of the Monasteries the Poor Law Act of 1601 decreed that such care should become the responsibility of individual parish councils – these also 'prescribed' occupation. The Industrial Revolution that began in the 18th century provides the background to and perhaps the cause of the breakdown of this system of care, leading as it did to massive mental as well as physical and social ill-health. Asylums were built, soon becoming overcrowded, and occupation was seen as of economic rather than therapeutic value. Mental illness came to be viewed as a divine punishment for sin - a cruel approach which was denounced by the 18th century pioneers of a new 'moral treatment': pioneers such as Phillippe Pinel in France and William Tuke in York, England, who banned physical restraint and advocated patience and gentleness in the treatment of the mentally ill. In 1838 the foundation of St. Andrew's Hospital in Northampton was based on this 'moral treatment', the first Medical Superintendent, Thomas Prichard, directing his staff to show *'forbearance, gentleness and a spirit of mildness, moderation and forgiveness, directed by a merciful and intelligent understanding'*.

Behind all this history is the continuing philosophy that occupation is a natural state and a pre-requisite of health, that people should be treated as individuals with differing needs and aspirations, and that occupation should be used as a therapeutic agent. At St. Andrew's Hospital in the 19th century, for example, it is clear that activities were being provided that were designed to help treat the resident patients – piano playing for the women, cricket for the men. Newspapers were delivered; a bagatelle table was bought; a pony-chaise was presented to the residents; dances were held regularly and a brass band played once a week in summer. Work on the hospital farm was provided and later, in about 1910, garden allotments for the residents were introduced.

The shift of focus in the early 20th century is thought to have been a result of two factors – the new Arts and Crafts movement and the effect of the First World War. The Arts and Crafts movement became very popular and emphasised the virtues of creative activities at the expense of previous hobbies such as music, farming, walking, reading, debating and chess.

Then in the First World War (and 20 years later the Second) it was realised that occupational therapy, which had long been used in psychiatric hospitals, also had a valuable place in rehabilitating the physically disabled and injured. Doctors and military leaders wanted to re-establish a workforce depleted by war, so treatment was driven by medical and military beliefs in the need to get the wounded and disabled servicemen back to work. People were classed as 'cases' and 'patients', their own occupational preferences not taken into account.

The other important part of the story behind occupational therapy as it emerged in the 20th century is the way in which society was evolving, finding it more socially acceptable for women to take up careers. Medical knowledge was expanding rapidly and the care of the sick became a more respectable profession - one which was eminently suited to women.

> **St. Andrew's Hospital**
> **School of Occupational Therapy**
> NORTHAMPTON
> *Under Medical Direction.*
>
> The course of training extends over a period of 2 to 3 years. Students are prepared for the full Diploma of the Association of Occupational Therapists only.
>
> Studies include Craft work at the Northampton School of Arts and Crafts; Lectures in Anatomy, Physiology, Psychology, Medical, Surgical and Mental Diseases which are given by the Medical Staff; Theory of Occupational Therapy and the organisation of Hospital Recreation under the supervision of trained Occupational Therapists; hospital practice in Mental, Orthopaedic and General Hospitals.
>
> Students must be not less than 18 years of age and have reached an educational level of School Certificate standard. A personal interview is essential.
>
> Fees: 30 guineas per annum. Scholarships of the value of £80 per annum are available for competition and are tenable during the second year.
>
> Hostel accommodation available for Junior Students.
>
> **For further particulars apply to the Director of Training:**
> **Mrs. E. J. Hombersley, B.A.**

1. Advertisement for the School 1948

When Dr. Casson opened the first School of Occupational Therapy in England in 1930, it was an attractive prospect for the young women who had grown up in the 1920s, many of them denied the opportunity of entering university, and eager to take advantage of their new independence. Dr. Casson had been inspired by a visit to the first American School in Boston, setting up her own residential clinic for female psychiatric patients and alongside that, a training school of occupational therapists. Three years later another school opened, in London; then the Edinburgh School in 1937. St. Andrew's began training students in 1941 and can therefore claim to be the fourth oldest in Britain and the third oldest in England.

In 1933 the government took steps to encourage the training of the new therapists, issuing a Memorandum on Occupational Therapy for Mental Patients. It recommended the introduction of 'Occupational Therapist' as a new grade of staff in the mental hospital, suggesting that one therapist would be needed for every 1000 beds, and that the different types of therapy should be classed as 'occupational', 'recreational' and 'social'. Occupational therapy would include work in a hospital's utility departments as well as handicrafts, and Recreational meant sport, physical fitness drills, walks and dancing.

The Board listed four advantages of the new therapy: firstly, it had a favourable influence on the patients' mental attitude, relieving boredom and depression and giving them hope. Secondly, it induced good habits, enabling them to learn cooperation and to control their behaviour. Thirdly, it promoted their physical health through exercise and a change of posture, and finally an improvement would be noted in the whole atmosphere of the hospital, through the social contact and the hope of recovery. The Memorandum also pointed out the economic value of the new therapy: there would be less destructive behaviour and a greater capacity for useful work. The benefits would even be felt by the public who would learn to stop regarding mental hospitals as closed units. The Memorandum's recommendation to introduce a new grade of 'occupational therapist' was of course highly significant. It gave the impetus for the establishment of more training schools to follow on from Dr. Casson's example.

At St. Andrew's Hospital the Medical Superintendent appointed in 1913, Daniel Rambaut, carried on supporting the use of activities to benefit the health and well-being of the patients. The 1930s saw the provision of all kinds of amusements and activities, ranging from bridge and billiards to hockey matches and bathing parties in the River Nene at Clifford Hill. However, it was not until Dr. Thomas Tennent's arrival as Medical Superintendent in 1938 that the provision of the profession of occupational therapy was put on a more organised footing.

Dr. Tennent had been Deputy Superintendent of the Maudsley Hospital in London and Assistant Physician in Psychological Medicine at King's College Hospital. The governors at St. Andrew's were delighted with his appointment and spoke of his 'high attainments and considerable clinical and administrative experience at the Maudsley and other hospitals'. He appointed Miss Violet Parry as the occupational therapist for the ladies in 1938, and Miss E. Platt in 1940. They were assisted by three staff called 'ladies' companions', two of whom were elderly sisters, the Misses O'Connell, who retired in 1945. An average of 62 ladies attended the occupational therapy sessions, held in the wards and sitting rooms. On the male side, Dr. Tennent realised the lack of male occupational therapists available in general and so he sent a male nurse, Mr. Chatfield, to the Maudsley Hospital to attend a course of instruction. The carpentry workshop was enlarged in 1939, having been created a few years previously, and the occupational therapy staff included two 'gentlemen's companions'.

By 1941 the hospital was of course already feeling the effects of war, not only in the bomb damage inflicted but in the nature of its clientele. In January and April of that year two bombs fell on the golf course and front lawn, causing damage to one of the wards, and a new 'Military Unit' was set up for the treatment of psychiatric casualties in the Women's Services. As many as 1443 women were treated in 1941. The number of male staff was diminishing because men were leaving to join the Services, although several retired staff were welcomed back to help out. The urgent shortage of doctors and psychiatrists meant that Dr. Tennent twice asked the hospital Board of Control for permission to allow him to employ foreign nationals. For instance, he knew that there was a number of eminent Austrian psychiatrists keen to work in Britain. His request was turned down at first in 1939, but finally granted in 1941.

This increase of tension and activity induced by the war, coupled with the shortage of staff, provides the background against which Dr. Tennent decided to train his own occupational therapists. It was nothing as dramatic as the founding of the School at Dorset House, Bristol, by Dr. Casson: In January of 1941 Dr. Tennent had received a letter from a nurse in Yorkshire, enquiring about the possibility of training as an occupational therapist at St. Andrew's. This was probably the catalyst which led him to approach the Northampton School of Art to see if they would cooperate by giving instruction in art and crafts. He had in mind that the course should extend over 12 months and cost a nominal fee of 3 guineas, with the student(s) living outside the hospital. He had the support of the hospital's Board of Control and so now had to find likely students for the new School. It is not clear whether the nurse from Yorkshire did in fact come down to Northampton, but Rosemary Vaughan (née Elmer) has provided her own vivid recollections of how she found herself becoming the very first student occupational therapist at St. Andrew's.

She was a local girl who had started a general art course at the School of Art in 1939 and had barely been there a year when the Principal, Mr. Fred Courtney, called her in to his office to ask if she would be interested in training at the new School at St. Andrew's. She admits that she didn't know what she wanted to do for a career and that occupational therapy didn't mean anything to her, but Mr. Courtney's description of the work sounded quite interesting. It even had the added advantage of forming part of the war effort, so she finally decided to start the course in 1941. Rosemary was soon joined by one of the other art students, Pauline Barnes (née Pickford), and then three more students arrived – Sylvia Roberts, April Scott-Watson and Norah Cochrane.

A scheme of training had been drawn up by Dr. Tennent and Mr. Courtney whereby crafts were taught at the Art College and medical subjects at the hospital, in the lecture room of the nurses' home. Pauline believes that initially Dr. Tennent proposed to issue a Certificate of Qualification from St. Andrew's, but the students quickly realised that it was the Diploma of the Association of Occupational Therapists (A.O.T.) that they would need in order to gain employment. They therefore brought pressure on Dr. Tennent to enable them to take the Association's examination, which he duly arranged.

Dr. Tennent clearly saw that in setting up a School he was furthering the progress of this new profession, of whose value St. Andrew's had for so long been deeply aware. Nevertheless he also saw the value of training therapists who would be useful aides while students, and possible future permanent members of staff. Even though his motives may have partly centred on the needs of his hospital, it is true to say that St. Andrew's, as a charitable trust, has always considered it an important part of its role to help and support the non-private sector of the health service. By subsidising the occupational therapy course of training, the governors knew they were indirectly benefiting patients both in their own hospital and in those other hospitals to which qualified therapists would subsequently be appointed. It was believed that there must be many suitable candidates deterred from training by virtue of the expensive fees that were normally charged. So the School's Committee of Management ensured that their own fees were set within a candidate's means and where necessary, grants were given. Thus, in 1942, two of the 2nd year students were given a grant of £80 p.a. each.

It must have been daunting for Rosemary and Pauline to enter the grounds of St. Andrew's Hospital and begin their training. Neither of them referred to the impression created by the beautiful surroundings and grand main building. Both recall the way in which every room was locked. Rosemary recalls, *'The first thing they did was give you a bunch of keys to let you in and out of all the wards, and that was it really. You were told to teach various crafts, and we had shadow boards on the walls for scissors etc .They were all checked against the boards at the end of a session and if there was a pair of scissors missing, the patients weren't allowed out until it was found. It was a wonderful experience, but we were absolutely in the dark. We went along on our own. We were based in Wantage House and literally started off from a cupboard with probably a few shoe boxes to put our bits and pieces in.'* The first piece of craft work done by the students was a macramé cord for their scissors, which was then attached to the belt of their uniform.

With no knowledge whatsoever of mental illness, Pauline remembers being given the keys to a sitting room and told to lock herself and Rosemary in with the patients. If they were in with the more severely affected patients on the top floor, they were accompanied by experienced staff, but she refloots that they were not trained to take basic precautions such as keeping in a corner of the room in order to be able to see the whereabouts of each patient. '*We ourselves had pairs of scissors which had to be supervised if anyone wished to use them, also materials and very small looms (which we had had no training in using). I have not forgotten the patient who was weaving a scarf. When the moment of truth came and the scarf was removed from the loom, I discovered to my horror that I had omitted to allow any wastage! All my skill was employed in the next little while persuading her that short scarves were 'in' that winter. I was at the same time terrified that I might have set her recovery back months! ... In the Back Wards, where all the worst patients were, we went armed with cardboard boxes containing mostly dishcloth cotton and large knitting needles ... One patient, I remember, insisted on increasing at each end of every row, so that we produced a series of triangular dishcloths.*'

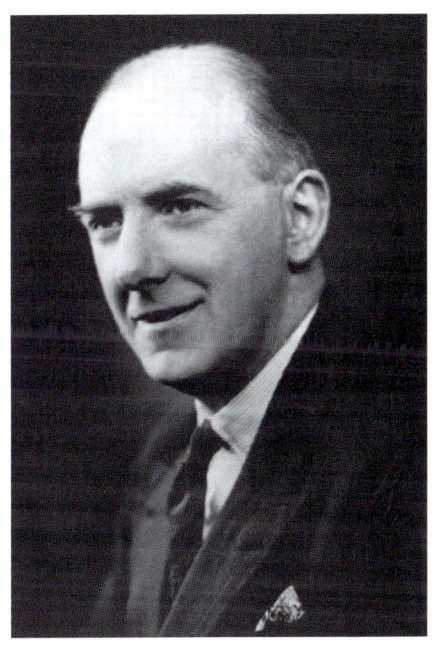

2. Dr. Tennent

It seemed particularly hard on the students that they were not allowed to see the patients' case histories. The reason given was that St. Andrew's was a hospital 'for the middle and upper classes' and the patients were private. They were paying considerable sums of money to attend the hospital, so to reveal their problems to the students was considered inappropriate. '*The idea seemed to be that the patients could do as they wished.*' It is interesting to compare the way in which the St. Andrew's students had to learn on the job, so to speak, and the method used at Dorset House. Dr. Casson was also known to throw prospective students in at the deep end in order to assess their suitability for the profession. Constance Owens (née Tebbit) recalls being assessed during a social evening with patients and later being left to her own devices in an acute ward. However, Dorset House was run as a kind of commune akin to the communal Utopias that were conceptualised in 19th century philosophy and earlier, with everyone contributing to the welfare of the whole. There were no sharp social or professional distinctions between members of staff and patients. The experience of being a student at St. Andrew's, the largest psychiatric hospital in Europe and a private one advertising itself for the upper and middle classes only, was inevitably different from the experience of studying under Dr. Casson.

At this time St. Andrew's owned several large Victorian villas in the grounds where elderly patients lived. Rosemary recalls how some of them were very clever, and all were from very wealthy families. *'I think that some of the families had put them there to get them out of the way, if you like. Perhaps they were being a bit of trouble to the family and they thought they'd send them to St. Andrew's to be looked after. They were pretty harmless.'* The students also became involved in treating the many Service people who had been admitted since the outbreak of war. They would give them peg rugs and weaving to do, encouraging the use of bright colours if they had depression or similar problems in order to lift their mood.

The training course was organised so that the students attended lectures at the hospital in the morning and crafts at the School of Art in the afternoon. The School of Art was in the building now forming Avenue Campus on St. George's Avenue and part of the University of Northampton. All the students had bicycles and cycled back and forth across the Racecourse to attend their various sessions. Medical lectures were given by Dr. Gibson, Major O'Connell and in the final year, Colonel Tennent. Both the latter wore army uniform, reflecting their military rank. The students were given experience in observing the new medical treatment, Electrically induced Convulsive Therapy (ECT). Great strides were being made in the treatment of schizophrenia. In 1938 Dr. Tennent had introduced the use of the drugs cardiazol and insulin, but it was a complicated technique, and in 1941 was replaced by ECT, said to be far less unpleasant for the patient. Rosemary, however, remembers feeling quite frightened at seeing the ECT being administered. *'They'd lie them on the bed, hold on to their limbs and put something in their mouth so they didn't bite their tongue. They'd give them these vast electric shocks and the patient would go into terrific spasms. After a time they'd come round and wouldn't remember a thing about it. They were quite frightened about having it done, but they didn't remember a thing.'* (The treatment was developed because psychiatrists had observed that some patients who had had a spontaneous epileptic fit showed improvement in their

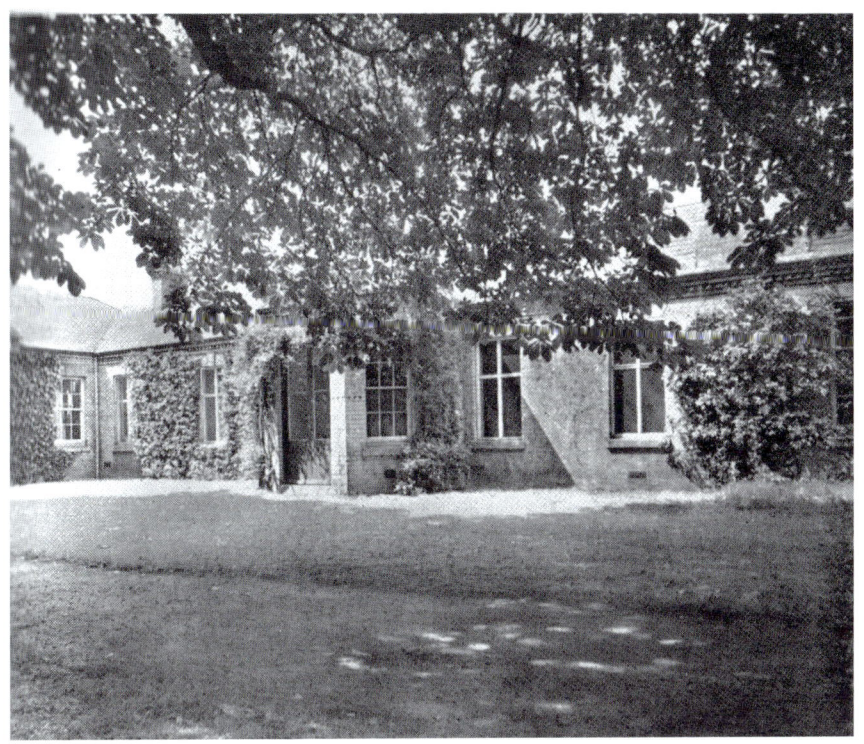

3. The School building 1950

mood. This led to fits being induced as a method of treatment for severe depression which did not respond to drug therapy.)

It must have seemed a totally different world in the School of Art. Not all crafts were taught there for Mr. Chatfield in the hospital woodwork shop near the main gates was able to teach the students carpentry. Patients working there were bemused at the sight of girls sawing wood. Pauline remembers having to fend off offers of help with her mortise and tenons.

The whole course was to cover two years and led to the award of the Psychological Diploma, being only related to occupational therapy for psychiatric patients. Orthopaedic training required an extra year at a suitably equipped School, and gave the dual qualification, meriting a whole £20 extra on an occupational therapist's annual salary.

In 1943 the School was recognised as an official training establishment under the A.O.T., and Dr. Tennent asked the governors for permission to engage an occupational therapist to be in charge of the School. Now in their second year, the students had been expressing concern that their syllabus was not covering the topics of Department Management and Approach to Patients. It was timely therefore that in July 1943 Dr. Tennent appointed Miss Mabel Thompson to run the Occupational Therapy department and teach the students the required syllabus. She was an American lady who had qualified at the Boston School. Although her stay was only relatively brief, her appearance made a lasting impression on the students. *'Clad in Dr. Kildare-style white, including white hat, white stockings and white shoes, she talked a lot about 'projects'. She did, it is true, put some order into our lives, but left rather a lot undone when, about six weeks before the Final Examinations, she threw up her hands, said it was all impossible and departed.'* Dr. Tennent was still searching for a replacement in May the following year.

Little is known about Miss Thompson, the lady in white, but she may well have played a part in inspiring her students with a fervent belief in the value of occupational therapy as a way of restoring the spirit as well as the body: In 1946 she sent in to the Journal of the AOT this lengthy quote of a statement made in 1919 by the novelist, John Galsworthy, at the Allied Conference on the After-Care of Disabled Men. It is almost a rallying cry for the new profession, and Miss Thompson suggested it should be in every occupational therapist's notebook: *'Restoration is at least as much a matter of spirit as of body, and must have as its central truth: - Body and spirit are inextricably conjoined. To heal the one without the other is impossible. If a man's mind, courage and interest be enlisted in the cause of his own salvation, healing goes on apace, the sufferer is re-made; if not, no mere surgical wonders, no careful nursing, will avail to make a man of him again. Therefore, I would say: 'From the moment he enters the hospital, look after his mind and his will; give him food; nourish him in subtle ways; increase the nourishment as his strength increases. Give him interest in his future. Light a star for him to fix his eyes on, so that, when he steps out of the hospital, you shall not have to begin to train one who for months, perhaps years, has been living, mindless and will-less, the life of a half-dead creature. A niche of usefulness and self-respect exists for every man however handicapped; but that niche must be found for him. To carry the process of restoration to a point short of this is to leave the cathedral without a spire. To restore him, and with him the future of our countries, that is the sacred work.'*

While Dr. Tennent was looking for a replacement for Miss Thompson, the students were greatly helped by the Principal of Dorset

House, Miss E.M. MacDonald, who heard of their plight and invited all five of them to her School (now re-located to Bromsgrove). Here they completed the required syllabus and were helped to pass their Finals. The practical craft side of the exams involved taking about forty samples of work up to Birmingham to be handed in as part of the final papers. Two of the girls obtained distinction in individual subjects, and one of them failed. St. Andrew's rewarded the successful candidates by paying their exam fees.

In 1944 the official recognition of the School helped the students financially, for the new 1944 Education Act meant that all students attending a degree course or one considered equivalent, were eligible for a Local Education Authority or Ministry award. The occupational therapy diploma qualified for the award. The increase in applications during the

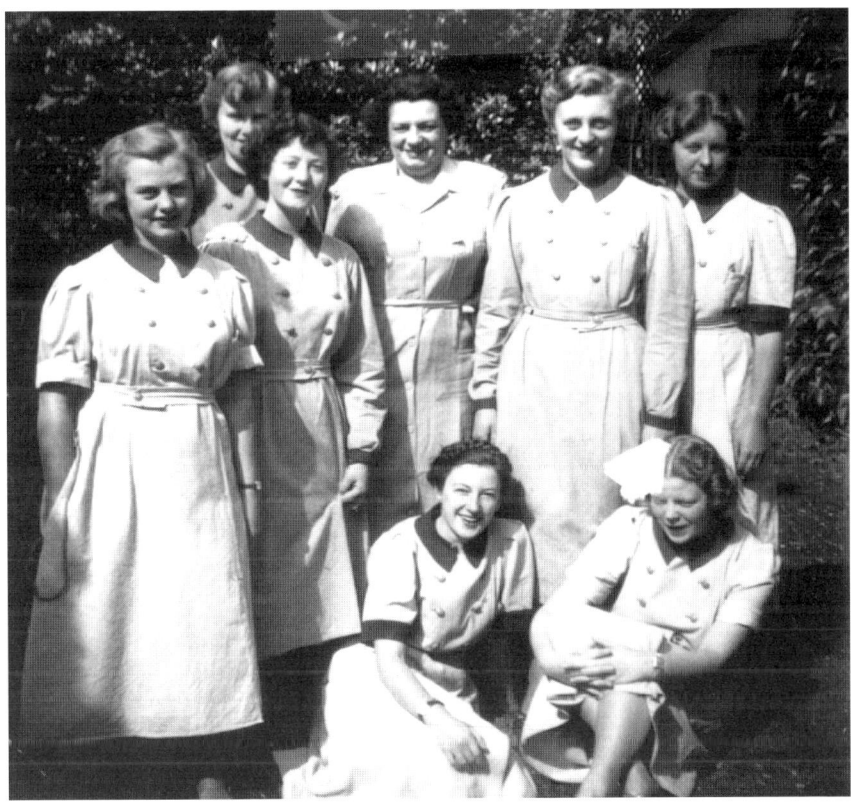

4. Violet Parry and some of the students, ca. 1951

late 40s and 50s can be seen as a result of this new source of funding. The applicants continued to be middle or upper class and female. They all came from private or grammar schools, which in the 1950s took only 10 – 25% of the country's pupils. The majority left school at the age of 15 - prior to 1951 the school-leaving age had been 14.

Subsequently the 1962 Education Act ensured that the L.E.A. award was mandatory for all full-time higher education students. It was to be means-tested and available regardless of the location of the course. The effect on the number of students was dramatic: in the 1920s some authorities had granted scholarships for university; by 1938 38% of undergraduates had either a scholarship or an assisted place; by 1951 the number had risen to 74%. The new mandatory awards in 1962 meant a huge expansion of the undergraduate population encouraged also by the growing affluence of the country – increasing prosperity leading to a greater demand for higher education. So with the new mandatory provision of grants, St. Andrew's tradition of subsidising its students' studies became less necessary.

To return to the early days of the St. Andrew's School: by 1943 the first group of students had completed the two year psychiatric course. Dr. Tennent worked to improve the facilities and organisation of the training and by 1944 seven students were attending the School. First and foremost, he was pleased to appoint Mrs Joyce Hombersley as Director of Training and Head Occupational Therapist. Mrs Hombersley had gained considerable experience at the Maudsley Hospital and abroad. Dr. Tennent felt great confidence in her leadership and reported that he looked forward to the School *'taking a leading position in the country'*.

He knew that he also needed to improve the physical facilities, ensure the ablest students be admitted and that hostel accommodation be provided. There was still not much competition as far as other Schools were concerned, with only three other Schools being open at the end of the war. By 1946 Dorset House had moved to Oxford and was housed in eighteen poorly heated Nissan huts and six brick huts. The London School was in an old Victorian house in Hampstead, run by two ladies, remembered as 'the aunts', one slim and elegant, the other small and round often with two dachsunds tucked under her arms. St. Loyes in Exeter was founded in 1945 under the auspices of St. Loyes Training Centre for Cripples; Liverpool would only open in 1947 and Derby in 1948.

Training for the new profession of occupational therapy was still in its infancy when Mrs. Hombersley arrived. In 1939 there were only 100

occupational therapists on the register of the A.O.T. in England. After the shut-down of courses in 1939, a steady expansion had resumed but there was still an acute shortage in 1944. Occupational therapy as a profession expanded very rapidly during the war, concentrating on the physical rehabilitation of injured Service people and developing specialised spinal injury units. Prior to this, the physical side had hardly moved on since the 'curative workshops' of World War I. This concentration led Mrs. Hombersley to lament the loss of groundwork in the psychiatric side of occupational therapy during the war years; she sent in a letter to that effect that was published in the Journal of the AOT in 1944. She had reviewed a paper by Drs. Sargeant and Slater on 'Physical Methods of Treatment in Psychiatry' where she noted their lack of confidence in the 'precise indications' of occupational therapy, and so she suggests that a more scientific and critical approach is needed '*if we are not to slip back 20 years and find ourselves damned once more with the 'Arty-Crafty' label. What seems to be needed is a certain amount of work on something like the following lines: -*
 a) *a group of patients receiving physical treatment together with strenuous Occupational Therapy.*
 b) *Control group receiving physical treatment but no Occupational Therapy.*
 c) *Group receiving Occupational Therapy but no physical treatment.*
 d) *Control group receiving no treatment of either kind.*
The patients in each group should be as nearly approximated as possible and the results tabulated after a period of say six months or a year. Detailed records of work periods, occupation given, patients' reactions to various types of work, etc. would be essential, and naturally very close co-operation from the Medical Officers in charge of the physical treatment would be necessary.'

Her fears were understandable, for the 1930s had seen tremendous activity and excitement as the profession began to establish itself. Medical and political interest had been stimulated, with the government calling for more posts and departments being set up in both physical and mental hospitals. The war had interrupted this process. Now that the war was over, the profession needed to redress the balance and ensure that clinicians, politicians and the general public understood the essence of what occupational therapy was all about.

A promotional leaflet published by the A.O.T. in the early 1950s refers to the fundamental misunderstanding that lay behind '*the growing tendency to distinguish between 'diversional therapy' as a term covering those types of work intended simply to raise morale and relieve boredom and 'occupational therapy' as meaning treatment directed to a more specific purpose.'* An editorial in the Journal of the Association of Occupational Therapy just before the end of the war stated the case: *'Terminology must be used with care – not "Diversional'* or *'Remedial', but local, specific, or general. All patients – physically and mentally ill – want to be <u>treated</u>. Who shall say that the exercise of a stiff elbow has greater remedial value than the relief of strain in a fear-filled mind, or that it is more therapeutic to mobilise stiff limbs than it is to mobilise fresh thoughts? The tendency during the war years has been to emphasise the physical aspect of occupational therapy at the cost of the psychological. We can make no greater mistake than to separate them.'*

This view was grounded in the original concept of the profession – one that is client-centred and aimed at enabling occupation which has meaning as well as, or despite, a curative focus. Joyce Hombersley's fears indicate how she herself was well aware of the shift which was taking place within the profession.

However, she had a new School to build up and a promising environment in which to carry out her task. Only a year before her arrival the first student at St. Andrew's had completed her qualification. Making it through those first two years had had the feeling of being part of an experiment: *'We were really just guinea pigs. I can feel the weight and hear the rattle of those keys still, when I go to bed at night.'*

Chapter 2

Foundations

Joyce Hombersley 1944 – 1957

1948 NHS established – Initial excitement over the new therapy fades after World War II – Shortage of therapists but only two more Schools open – 1948 new Teacher's Diploma in Occupational Therapy – 1955 first use of phrase 'Activities of Daily Living' (ADL) – New tranquillising drugs in mental health service enable more rehabilitation.
Huge demand for places at St. Andrew's School after the War – 1954 new syllabus combines Physical and Psychological Diplomas – 1955 first thesis on occupational therapy accepted at a British university.

'There appears to be a great future for the profession, which is becoming acknowledged as a valuable medical auxiliary service and an essential link in the progressive treatment of those individuals who are so unfortunate as to suffer from disease or injury with all their attendant evils, physical, psychological, economic and social.' So runs the A.O.T.'s promotional leaflet in 1951. However, Joyce Hombersley's concern for the future of the profession seems to have been well founded. Despite all the energy that was released on social improvements after the war, the provision of occupational therapy facilities seemed to slow down, at least in civilian hospitals. Reasons suggested have been a lack of funds, a lack of qualified therapists, and a lack of medical supervisors. Also the profession was not promoting itself adequately to explain what valuable goals it could achieve. There may even have been a certain post-war apathy setting in by the 1950s.

There was no uniform government plan to utilise occupational therapists, with perhaps too many different bodies being responsible for them – the Ministry of Health, the Ministry of Labour, local authorities, voluntary societies. It was too early in the profession's life for a proper survey to have been carried out into the needs of the various groups of the population who could benefit from the therapy. In 1958 there were still only 1453 occupational therapists employed in the hospital service in England and Wales. In 1952 the view had been expressed that occupational therapists were wrongly distributed, by far the majority being employed to work with in-patients. Overall one third worked in physical rehabilitation and were mostly located in London, while two thirds had posts in mental hospitals.

Despite the shortage of qualified staff only one new school opened after Derby in 1948 – this was Botley's Park in 1949, based in Chertsey, Surrey, a home for people with special needs. No school opened in the 1950s at all, with the Glasgow School being founded in 1962.

In the physical field occupational therapists concentrated on restoring physical independence to women, children and the elderly, and were largely excluded from the process of resettlement into paid work. The government was spending money on aids such as home helps, day nurseries and meals on wheels instead of paying occupational therapists to make the housewife more independent with the aid of gadgets and adaptations. Nowadays the phrase, 'Activities of Daily Living', is familiar, and people talk about ADL to refer to the various aids that now exist for daily tasks. However, the phrase was only first used officially in 1955 in a government publication, 'Services for the Disabled', and in actual fact there were few ADL available commercially. In the 1950s most were being devised and made in occupational therapy departments by the therapists themselves.

In the area of mental health, occupational therapists were beginning to see the effects of the new drugs which were now in use. Anti-anxiety and anti-psychotic drugs such as largactyl and chlorpromazine were making it possible to rehabilitate disturbed patients who would previously have only been receptive to palliative treatment. Chlorpromazine was developed in 1950 and led to a breakthrough in drug treatment in psychiatry. It is said to have revolutionised the management of cases of mania and schizophrenia by producing remission of the symptoms. This would clearly help further the use of occupational therapy in mental hospitals. Some of these patients could even be discharged into the community, and many were found to be suffering more from the effects of institutionalisation than mental illness. The mental hospital population did in fact reach a peak in 1954, after which it declined. New developments were also evident in the discussions about the possibilities for occupational therapy outside the realm of the hospital, such as the provision of training during convalescence, and industrial workshops for those with special needs. In general, in the 1950s the main areas of occupational therapy, apart from psychiatry, were cerebral palsy, poliomyelitis, tuberculosis, rehabilitation and resettlement.

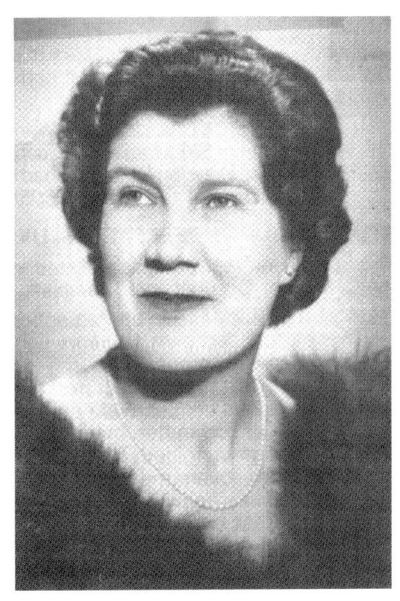

The A.O.T., formed in 1936, realised the need to train more therapists and that it was not just schools that were required – teachers were needed to work in these schools. So in 1948 a Teacher's Diploma was inaugurated, comprising a two year in-service course. The Association had produced the first syllabus for training students back in 1938. It remained largely unchanged for 40 years. The Preliminary Examination required a knowledge of anatomy, physiology, psychology and first aid. In all cases in the Final Examination students studied departmental management, general medicine and surgery, and applied psychology. Then according to specialisation they would either study psychiatry, psychopathology and occupational therapy applied to psychiatric conditions, or advanced anatomy and physiology, physical medicine and orthopaedics, and the application of occupational therapy to physical conditions. On top of these academic subjects, an advanced knowledge was required of two basic crafts and a good grounding in eight minor ones, together with practical experience with patients for 32 or 36 weeks (according to age).

5. *Joyce Hombersley*

The preliminary and final exam papers for 1952–4 (see Appendix) reveal the rigour of the syllabus, some of the medical modules being taken to a level said to be the equivalent of the first MD doctor's exams. The students found that they had to learn a lot of the Medicine and Surgery by rote, some finding the course extremely hard. *'Everyone had a Gray's Anatomy, which was very expensive and passed down from one year to the next.'* Being such a new profession, the types of textbook available were still not always suitable. Eventually, for example, a more elementary anatomy textbook was brought out more suited to occupational therapists' and nurses' requirements. *'You can see how we were hammered with our anatomy exam. They really got mad if you couldn't do it. You used to have to draw it with chalk on the board ... In the second year we took an exam on psychopathology which was horrendous.'*

In the early days some students had been accepted without their having matriculated, (which was the equivalent of having two A-levels). So on top of their studies they had to work to matriculate in English. *'We really worked very hard and tried very hard.'* Fortunately for Mrs. Hombersley. some of her students had a very positive enthusiastic attitude to their studies, and her little annual talk to the first years may not always have been necessary. She would announce that she most definitely was not running a pre-marriage course. Her fears concerning the attitude of some of her students turned out to be well-founded. In the 1944 intake, two out of the six failed to finish the course – one girl left at the end of the probationary term and the other only attended in the first year when she chose to. *'Mrs. H. thought it would be a good idea if she left.'* Another of the early students is remembered with some affection for her lack of motivation and sense of guilt. She received a grant because she was retraining after a period in the armed forces, and admitted to feeling very guilty about it: *' "They keep giving me money!" She couldn't understand it.'* Other girls in later years, even in the mid 50s, simply dropped out because they got married: *'When you got married in those days, that was it. You didn't work; you certainly didn't go to college. You weren't expected to continue.'*

For those who were enthusiastic about their chosen career their first post could be very challenging and exciting because it was in the days when departments were still being opened. Your first post could easily be to set up a new occupational therapy department, as happened to Pauline Barnes and Kay Kennedy at Manfield Orthopaedic and St. Crispin's respectively.

In 1946 Dr. Tennent was pleased to state in his annual report that the School could now train students for the full Diploma of the A.O.T., although orthopaedic training had to be undertaken at Manfield and was still optional. Then in 1953 the School could announce that the majority of the students now remained for the third year to gain the physical qualification (and hence the full Diploma). In 1954 the syllabus was revised. No longer could students opt to do just the physical or psychological side, and the structure of the course was overhauled and made more relevant to occupational therapy in practice. As a result of the new syllabus the St. Andrew's School decided to stop using the Northampton School of Art and carry out all the technical / craft training at the hospital. Dr. Tennent wrote: *'The changes in syllabus have necessitated a new approach to the teaching of practical subjects. Hope-*

Two Days at an Occupational Therapy TRAINING SCHOOL

The Occupational Therapy training course lasts for three years, and at least one year is spent in practical work in various types of hospitals. Here, to give the reader some slight idea of the compass of a student's work, is a timetable for two days at a typical training school.

First Day

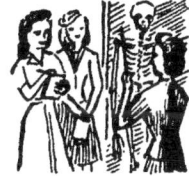

Morning Lecture : Anatomy and Physiology.

Modelling Class.

Lecture : General medicine and surgery.

Afternoon : Rug-making Class.
Lecture : Orthopædics.

Second Day

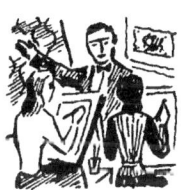

Morning Lecture : Psychiatry.

Weaving Class.

Afternoon Lecture :
Departmental management.

Design Class.

Lecture : Occupational therapy applied to psychological or physical conditions.

6. Timetable from the 1940s

fully it will be possible to link the practical, academic and clinical training far more closely by this method.'

Three large rooms on the top floor of the gentlemen's side of the hospital were equipped as craft rooms. The level of craftsmanship remained high, but no longer did the students have to reach the exacting standards of the Art School teachers, who were teaching the City and Guild syllabus. *'We had a horrible teacher up there. Her one favourite phrase was "It's not good enough". So you spent half your time undoing the stuff. It all had to be absolutely perfect.'* Students remember having to make elaborate toys; one produced a rocking horse and one a scale model of a theatre with stage, pulling curtains, footlights and wings.

For many years the first practical task given to the first years was to make a scissor cord using macramé. Needlework progressed to much larger projects as the students had to learn to weave a whole rug and a length of tweed. *'The rug rooms were in the attics and we used to try to arrange to go together because it was quite spooky when we were there at night. Getting back again, there weren't many lights in the grounds, but we had been used to using a torch in the war ... We did spinning there as well, quilting, smocking ...'* One of the looms was reputed to have woven the velvet used for Queen Victoria's wedding dress. Work on the large looms involved groups of two or three working together, using the same colour for their warp, but it took a long time. It was more fun to work on one of the smaller looms where one of the favourite creations was a tartan scarf. However, some girls did huge quantities of weaving – one even did enough to make the curtains of her first house.

Carpentry, basketry and leatherwork were usually done on Saturday mornings in the male patients' workshop. In the 1940s and 50s Northampton had many shoe factories where off-cuts of leather could be purchased, and students might be sent to buy their own pieces. In those days such an errand might expose an innocent 18 year old to more than she bargained for: *'She came back full of indignation and said, "It was a dreadful place. There was a whole wall with calendars of naked women." Of course you forget just how straight-laced the 50s were.'*

A wide array of woodwork pieces were made, ranging from cigarette boxes to an oak bench and a cupboard; one girl even made a real boat. *'The examiners who used to come round to look at our work were always absolutely amazed because the standards were so high and we made some wonderful things ... Our leatherwork was amazing too. The examiner said, "Of course, this has been done by a machine". "I promise you it hasn't! I stitched every stitch"... I did a red goatskin clutch bag which I still have now.'*

In the third year the clinical application of these creative skills could be brought to the fore, at times making a deep impression on the surgeons, still fairly unfamiliar with what occupational therapy could achieve. One former student remembers a patient who had had all his right hand fingers and thumb severed in an accident with a circular saw. As a student she had to try to make his palm malleable so he could

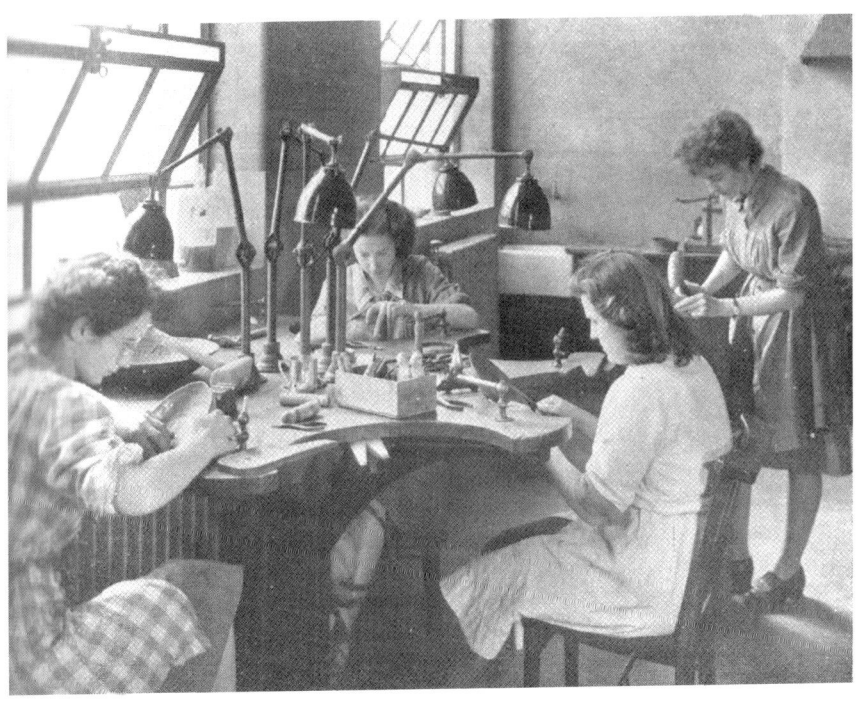

7. Light Metal Workshop ca. 1950

grip things. '*I made something like a glove with wire extensions inside so he could bend them and actually pick things up. We played drafts or solitaire or a card game so he had to pick things up. The end result was that he could hold a steering wheel and open door knobs ... The surgeon asked me what I'd been doing with the man's hand and I took the glove along to show him. He was quite enthralled by this ... It was my idea.'*

The amount of academic, practical and also clinical work that the students had to fit into their time necessitated a long working day. During the first year there were three sessions – morning, afternoon and evening from 5 – 6pm, the latter session being devoted to lectures. The other sessions were either practical or clinical. In the second year the greater part of one term was spent on clinical practice and the other term on practical work. The third term was taken up by exams. St. Andrew's was able to place students in a variety of local hospitals – Creaton TB Sanatorium, Manfield Orthopaedic Hospital, the Hospital of St. Cross, Rugby, Thorpe Hall Rehabilitation Centre, Peterborough, and St. Crispin's mental hospital.

Although 'Activities of Daily Living' were not officially spoken of until 1955, students from as early as 1945 remember being encouraged at Manfield to think about how patients would cope with their physical disabilities when they got home. A kitchen environment on the wards was not however provided until several years later. By 1953 the School was proud to announce that their third year students were being placed in no less than 14 different hospitals in the region.

During the 1950s the government began to try to organise the supply and demand of training and qualifications not just for occupational therapists but for all the Professions Supplementary to Medicine (PSMs). It was not however until 1960 that an Act of Parliament was passed to facilitate this. After the establishment of the National Health Service in 1948 attention had been more focused on the conditions of service of NHS employees. This was dealt with by the Whitley Council of the Health Service during the late 1940s. As far as St. Andrew's Hospital was concerned, they were able to remain outside the nationalisation process. Dr. Tennent announced in 1948 that permission had been granted to function outside the NHS, although some beds would be reserved for NHS patients. It was thought that independent management had the advantage of encouraging a progressive outlook and approach and could only serve to benefit psychiatry in general.

Amid this time of organisational and medical changes Joyce Hombersley's fears for the profession became even more significant. Along with many other occupational therapists she wanted a more scientific and critical attitude towards occupational therapy in order to avoid slipping back 20 years. After the war people did begin writing about the value of being able to measure improvement in joint mobility, for instance. They tried also to show improvements, for example, in the re-socialisation of victims who had been badly burned, or the mental health

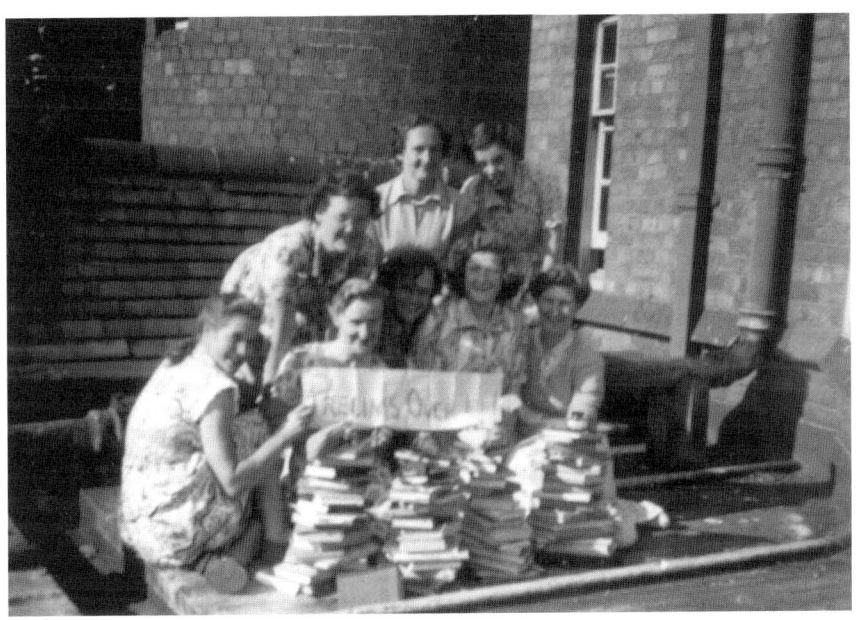

8. Prelims over! 1952

of children at play who were suffering from neuroses. The A.O.T. were of course aware of the need for research on the value of occupational therapy. It knew it had to act to support and defend the profession and raised the money to set up a Fellowship Fund. In 1947 the first Industrial Fellowship for 'Research into the Scope and Applications of Industrial Work' was awarded. Money, however, ran short and research became a reqular item on the agenda of the Council, who strove to raise sufficient funds in order to offer support. It was not until 1955 that the first thesis on occupational therapy was accepted for a degree at a British university. This was at Oxford University, and the candidate, Miss Mary Macdonald; her subject, 'The development of certain therapeutic services, their interrelationship and their place in the social framework. The effect of these factors on recruitment, selection and training of personnel'.

Back in 1944, when Joyce Hombersley was faced with the task of building up the St. Andrew's School, it is unlikely that her students had thoughts of research on their mind. They were mostly fresh out of school and just keen to embark on a career that promised a good future and called for students with a well rounded personality, good with their hands and good with people. One of the promotional leaflets of this period reads: '*In addition to the ability to do or to learn several crafts, a knowledge of music and/or folk dancing is helpful.*' The A.O.T.'s own leaflet states that *'Personal integrity and the power of winning and retraining the confidence of the patient are perhaps the most important (requirements for a good occupational therapist). Sympathy, tactfulness and good powers of observation are desirable qualities, especially if when linked to a cultural background and wide interests, they are manifested in an ability to arouse and stimulate similar interests in others. But the keystone of all such work must be a genuine interest in the patient as an individual, and a sense of service not only to that patient but to the community as a whole.'* Added to this the St. Andrew's School prospectus suggests *'a high degree of mental and general physical health is essential. Accordingly, a medical certificate of fitness must be furnished by a physician.'*

In 1951 the Association was recommending a required minimum educational standard of one A-Level in English, English Literature or History and four O-Levels, of which three should be English Language, a Science, and a Fine Art or Craft subject. Also, in view of the nature of the work of an occupational therapist, a diversity of interests was suggested as important for success. It was therefore also recommended that applicants should have continued with some form of physical education and with some extra-curricula activity throughout their school career.

Selecting prospective students was done with great care, everyone being offered an interview. Twelve students had been enrolled in 1944 at St. Andrew's, numbers being limited by the lack of space. Dr. Tennent had explained in his report for 1945 that the demand for places was 'enormous'. The School was housed in a series of rooms in a brick building backing on to the Billing Road near the main gates. It stood in its own garden and was separated from the hospital by bomb damage. One year later, in 1945, Dr. Tennent had obtained a former military hut at the cost of £100, so they were then able to increase the student intake to 18 or 20. The hut came to be used partly for students' craft work and partly for work with male patients. The existing large workshop for male patients was used for students' woodwork, basketry and leatherwork. Lectures still took place in the lecture room in the nurses' home.

In his reports to the hospital's Board of Control, Dr. Tennent reflected the nationalistic concern of the time. Preference was to be given as far as possible to girls who had been serving in the armed forces. He also commented that the current intake were all of British nationals. A few months earlier the Board had been reluctant to accept an application from a German refugee already training in mental nursing. They had only agreed to this under pressure from the Committee dealing with the

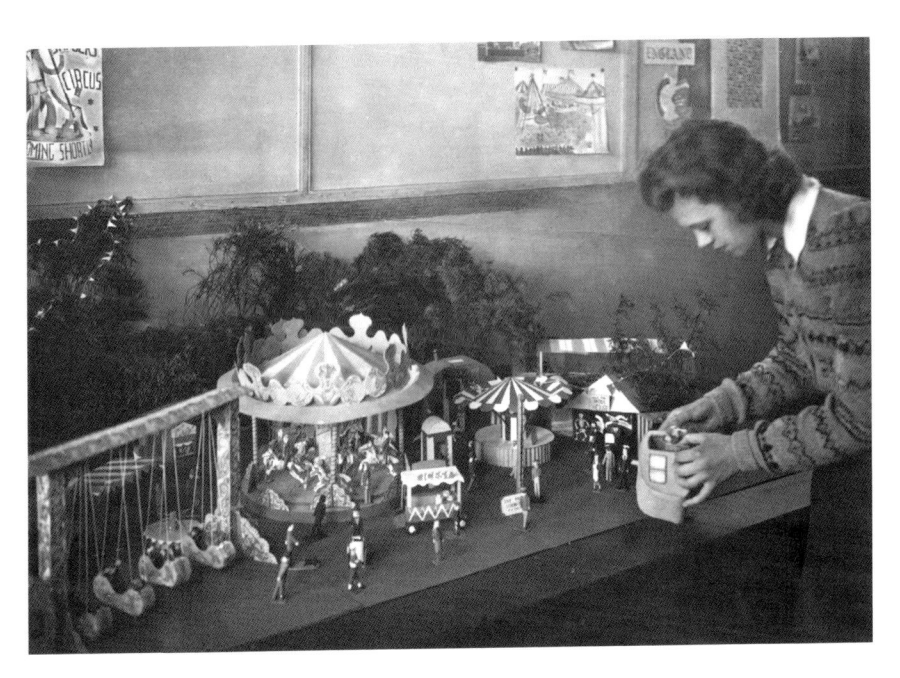

9. Toy Making 1950s

Refugees and the British Red Cross, and only after the suggestion from Dr. Tennent that these bodies be informed that firstly, the School must give preference to British students, and secondly, only one non-British student should be admitted, who would not be eligible for a grant from the hospital.

The increase in student numbers meant the scholarship fund was over-stretched. In late 1945 it was decided to award seven £80 annual grants to the second years, one for the most outstanding first year and six for students who in Dr. Tennent's opinion required help to complete their studies. Although the demand for places was said to be huge in the mid to late 1940s, in 1944 Joyce Hombersley and Dr. Tennent still found it necessary to seek out suitable students in the Northampton School of Art. One student from 1944 recalls how her mother had sent for the St. Andrew's School prospectus while she was attending an art course at the College. She remembers how Dr. Tennent and Mrs. Hombersley had come to talk to some of the art students. '*I was fetched out of a life class and I gathered they were interviewing me to see whether I was the correct sort of student to do occupational therapy. That was the first thing I knew about it. Dr. Tennent said finally, "Well she seems to be a fairly mature 17 year old" and Mrs. Hombersley said, "Yes. You would like to do occupational therapy, wouldn't you?" I said, "Yes", and went away to find out what it was.'*

An interview in 1955 suggests that Dr. Tennent had perfected a rather subtle approach to selection. The student in question remembers how strange it had seemed at the time: '*The funny thing was he didn't ask me anything else other than about playing hockey ... What position I played and why I had that position. I think my father thought 'What kind of a set-up is this?' But really he was asking what your passions were. Playing centre half, your job is to distribute play. You could be an attacker. You could be a defender. So you can be anywhere on the pitch and I quite liked that. I thought afterwards, maybe there is something in that. I think it was quite clever really.*' On the other hand other students have suggested that the interest shown in their sporting prowess was more straightforward. '*The only reason I got a place was because I have been keen on sport since I was a little girl, and it got me a place!*'

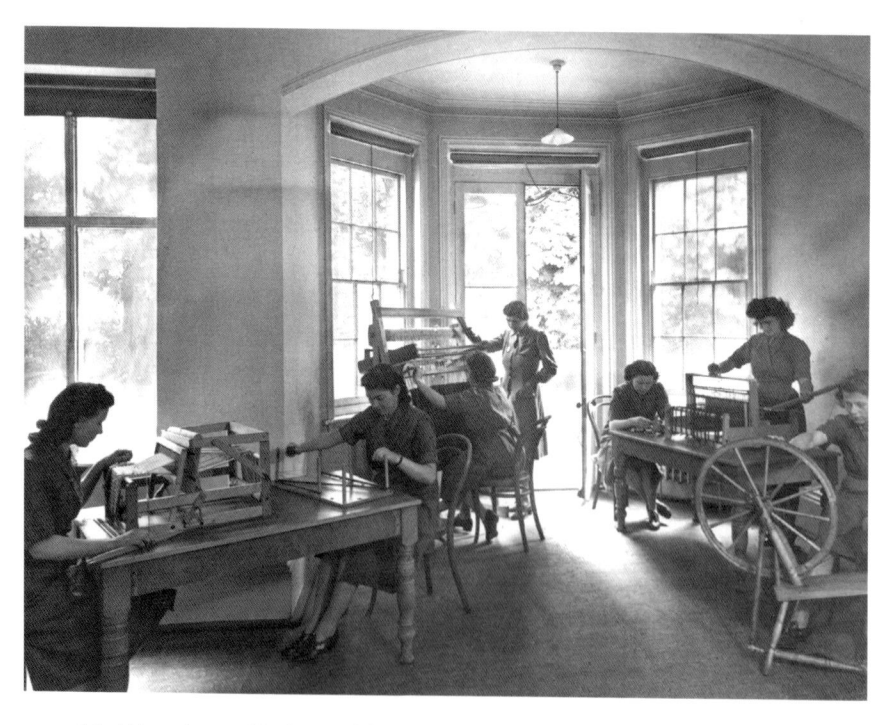

10. Weaving with Joyce Hombersley (in the background) ca.1947

For all the active promotion that was being done by the A.O.T., knowledge of the profession did not seem to be filtering down through the usual channels. Several past students recall finding out about occupational therapy from a member of their family or a perceptive forward-thinking teacher at school. *'The junior art mistress – her daughter was an occupational therapist. She must have thought that because of the science and art mixture, I might well fit into it ... She very kindly invited me to her home to meet her daughter and show me what she did. I never changed from that moment on.'*

Almost all of the past students who have contributed their memories enjoyed their time at the School and remember Mrs. Hombersley with great affection and admiration. On her arrival it was thought that her stay would be temporary, but she remained at St. Andrew's for thirteen years, 'developing the activities in the hospital and the training of the students in an exceptional manner'. She is remembered as an incredibly good teacher and a very human sort of person. *'Everybody loved her.'* She would talk to her students about a vast array of subjects, partly about life, partly on occupational therapy, partly on what was going on in the School (on which she always seemed very well informed, particularly on the various student misdemeanours). She was Scottish and had been married to an officer in the Indian army. During the war he had died from appendicitis in the middle of the desert, so Joyce was sent home with her baby son, Bill, on a troopship with all the hatches battened down The passengers had not been allowed on deck for about five weeks. She used to tell the story of how they had been held up for several days in the Bay of Biscay with the water running out and sanitary conditions generally deteriorating. Having finally landed up in the north of Scotland, she had had to get herself, her baby and all her luggage down to Bristol. *'She was certainly a redoubtable lady ... She could be quite imperious, but at the same time great fun.'*

Her rather glamorous appearance made a lasting impression: *'Always in her twinsets and tweeds ... Strange that it should be her red fingernails that stick in the memory ... At the St. Andrew's Day Ball and the annual garden party - Mrs. Hombersley, resplendent in dark silk splashed with poppies, a black straw hat, elbow-length kid gloves she had made herself, and the inevitable cigarette holder.'* One student recalls her bringing a black poodle, Benji, to class; another, how she had a habit of chain smoking even when lecturing. She had a house in Northampton to which some of her favourite students were invited to Sunday afternoon tea. Some resented the fact that she seemed to have her favourites, but others accepted the situation and admired Mrs. H. all the same. If they were shy, she was always sympathetic and encouraging.

Some of her sayings have inspired and stayed with her students all their lives: '*She always used to say, "We're only a small profession and you have to have the courage of your convictions. If you think something is right, you've got to have the courage to stand up for it." I can hear her voice saying that in my head even now ... I carried that all the way through – all the times when something was a bit difficult and "may be I'll just leave it": "You must have the courage of your convictions." I can hear her saying that quite clearly.*'

Poem from the 1940s

There's such a lot to learn about
With muscles, bones and joints
Their origins, insertions
And all their different points.
How can I learn them off by heart
And keep them in my head.
I wish I had a notebook here
To look them up instead.

The doctor bullies me and tries to
Tell me off if I forget.
He'd soon be lost without his pile
Of notes and book, I bet.
'Come up and draw a clavicle
With all its salient parts.'
So she creeps up to the blackboard
And nervously she starts.

'No, no, that's wrong, that will not do
That origin is bad!
If you do not get it this time you
Will make me very mad.
How can Pectoralis Major lie
Posterior to the rest?
Why don't you concentrate and
Try to do your best.?'

Poor student she is downcast,
She is weary, she is – blank,
For she can't remember anything
And for that she has to thank
The harshness of the doctor for
He looks so grim and stern
That she tries to guess at all the things
She hadn't time to learn.

Anne Dickens (Ridgeway)

Chapter 3

Work, Rest and Play

Joyce Hombersley 1944 – 1957 (cont.)

Students' uniforms – The hostels at Lowood and Rheinfelden – Social life in the 1950s – The Ball and the Eligibles Book – Entertaining the patients – Joyce Hombersley continues to encourage use of wide variety of occupations, not just crafts.

In these early days of the School there were two practical problems which had to be addressed – what would the students wear and where would they live? It is not clear when the uniform was introduced – certainly by about 1950 students were having to wear a grey double breasted thick cotton overall with long sleeves and scarlet collar and cuffs. The proliferation and tightness of the eleven buttons are still remembered with horror. *'There was no way you could get your hand in if the buttons were done up. There were three down the sleeves and then it was double breasted, and a couple on the belt ... The starched uniforms had to be peeled apart on their return from the hospital laundry and then you had to add the eleven buttons.'* Red shoes in the 1960s were a very popular accessory to the uniform.

The college scarf, grey with turquoise and red stripes, was much coveted but only awarded at the end of the probationary first term. One group of about six students felt so aggrieved at not being able to go home at Christmas sporting their own scarf like all their old school friends, that they decided to burn the midnight oil and make their own – in true occupational therapy fashion. *'We borrowed a scarf – we pinched one from the pegs where everybody hung their scarves when we went to dine at the nurses' home, took it down to Adnitt's (now Debenhams), matched the colour up, bought lengths of blue, grey and scarlet, put the scarf back, came back, cut all this up into strips and sat burning the midnight oil with a little tiny sewing machine so that we had scarves to go home with at*

Christmas. It took forever. It was a constant shift. The stripes had to go in a certain order. The funny thing was, when we held them up they twisted, but we had them for quite a long time.'

In January 1947 first year students could be accommodated in a villa in the hospital grounds that had been made into a hostel. It proved so popular that a Victorian house was bought on the Billing Road opposite the main gates, and equipped as a second hostel. Second years had to find their own 'digs' in town, although by 1950 they were able to live in 62a Billing Road. The hostels were in the charge of a warden, Mrs. Thomas, who was described by Dr. Tennent as 'efficient and sympathetic'. It must have been a hard task to look after dozens of 18-19 year old girls. In 1951 the total number of students at the School was 56.

'Lowood' and 'Rheinfelden' were the lovely villas which by 1953 had become hostels for the first and second years respectively, and which figure so prominently in past students' reminiscences. (In actual fact, Rheinfelden is said to have been used for the first years as early as 1950.) They are by and large remembered with affection despite or even because of the strict rules imposed by the various wardens – Mrs. Thomas, followed by Miss Woodall. Miss Woodall had come from a boys' boarding school where she had been matron to 12-14 year old boys. *'She was a tiny little thing and used to have platform soles on her shoes, with high heels. She was like a fairy, she was so small – gingery hair and very precise.'* Lowood still stands on the Avenue, off Cliftonville Road, now used by Social Services, but Rheinfelden was pulled down in the 1960s to be replaced by a block of flats on the corner of Cliftonville Road and Billing Road. It had only been used for three years because it was not really suitable for student accommodation and became a hostel for domestic staff. The villa was one of the elaborate turreted houses of which a few examples can still be seen along the north side of the Billing Road. It had been built by a diamond merchant after he had taken his wife on honeymoon down the Rhine and been inspired by the castles along the Rhine gorge. In 1956 the second year students moved out of Rheinfelden into Kingswood, almost opposite Lowood, and now no longer standing, replaced by a modern office building. In that year the School also acquired the Red House on the hospital's Moulton Park estate north of the town (the site of the present university). It became the hostel for the third years and was conveniently placed for students doing a clinical placement at Manfield Orthopaedic Hospital.

For the students in the hostels near St. Andrew's all meals were provided in the nurses' home, which was down a slippery path in the sunken area beyond the front lawns (now taken up by a 1980s housing estate). Rationing was still in place in the early 50s and the teas consisted only of bread and butter and a portion of plain cake. By 1953 past students recall the addition of jam and cheese – *'a real slab of yellow cheese'.* The canteen was also offering biscuits with the mid-morning coffee – food which students hadn't seen during the war. *'We*

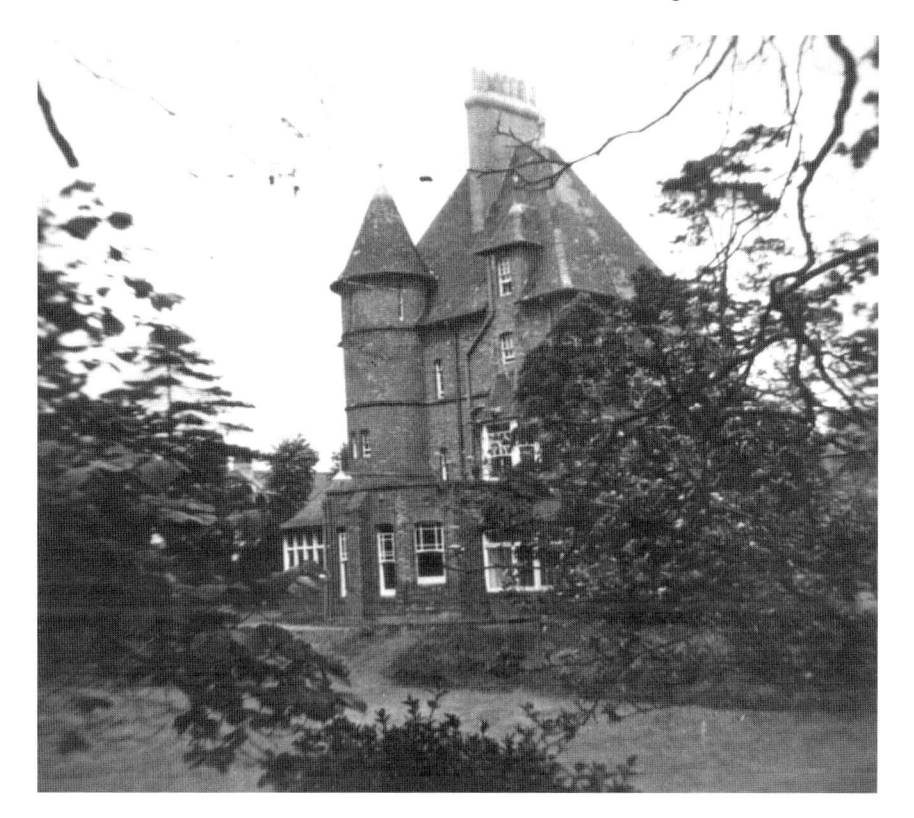

12. Rheinfelden student hostel 1949

used to have tea in the morning and coffee in the evening, but it was the same urn, so it all tasted the same really.' In the canteen there were some staff with learning disabilities – *'I shouldn't think any of us have forgotten Florrie. She used to come in with plates down her arm, and as she served they'd fall off down the table. We'd catch one or two.'* Sometimes there was a plague of ants and the students would know to bang the bread hard on the table to get rid of the ones lurking in the loaves. One past student remembers always being hungry on account of all the cycling backwards and forwards to the Art School and having lectures from 5 – 6pm (when she often fell asleep). Baked beans on toast was a favourite supplement to their diet. *' 'Uncle Tom' used to have a* corner shop across the Billing Road, down one of the side streets. He had all sorts in his shop – it looked like it hadn't been disturbed for ages, but we felt fairly safe with tins of baked beans which we ate in serious amounts. We were always "just going over to Uncle Tom's" to get chocolate or something like that – especially at exam time.'

Apart from memories of being hungry, there are several stories about the cold in the hostels. The students took it in turns to stoke the coke boiler every evening to keep the heating and hot water going. 'Everybody would shout at you if there was no hot water because you let the boiler go out. It was a real pig to light.' Stoking the boiler was one of the housekeeping duties for which each student was responsible for one week. One of the maids in the hostel was Rhona, who did the cleaning and made the beds. 'When you were on housekeeping duty you had to let Rhona in first thing in the morning – at 8 o'clock. There was a padlock and chain (on the hospital side gates). We used to all wear duffle coats, so you'd put your duffle coat over your pyjamas and go and open the gate. I remember saying to her on many occasions,"Rhona, I'm sure you could climb over these gates." We had to get milk in a jerry can from the nurses' home and a loaf so we could have something to eat in the evening … By the end of the week you'd just got into the habit of what you were supposed to be doing – the times you'd come back and had forgotten the loaf. You'd just get into the swing of it but then it was the next person's turn.' If the water was kept hot, three or four girls could have a bath each evening. There was a rota – 'so no luxurious soaking or someone would be banging on the door. There was a lot of trade in baths – if you were quick you could nip into a bath after a friend and do the same in reverse on *your* legitimate night.' There were only two bathrooms per hostel, and the bedrooms were furnished in an austere Victorian style, usually for four girls. '*Iron hospital beds with starched sheets and heavy wool blankets; lino on the floor with a small mat beside each bed, only one bedside lamp per room, two chests of drawers and one wardrobe for all to share*' – the memory is etched firmly on one student's mind.

Of course most of the stories remembered from this time centre on the various social activities. In the 1948 article promoting the School in the Journal of the A.O.T., Mrs. Hombersley mentions a 'flourishing student society', but it has not been mentioned by any past students. The system of college mums was in place in the mid-50s whereby a student wrote to a particular new girl before her arrival and helped her settle in, taking her round the various student haunts in town. Sometimes, with so much craft work to prepare, evenings were happily spent in the sitting room where a fire would be blazing and most students would be sitting doing something creative. One past student recalls evenings enjoyed listening to the radio: *'We had a battery operated radio and we couldn't afford the batteries very much. We used to have to save the batteries so we could listen to the Goons. You had to switch it off during the musical interlude to save the batteries for the second half.'* The Repertory Theatre was a favourite destination, plays usually changing once a week. The hard wooden terraced benches in 'the gods' only cost a shilling (5p), and well organised students would walk down to the theatre clutching a pillow to sit on. The seating arrangements might even be improved on if your friend sat behind you and let you lean against her legs, swapping over of course in the interval.

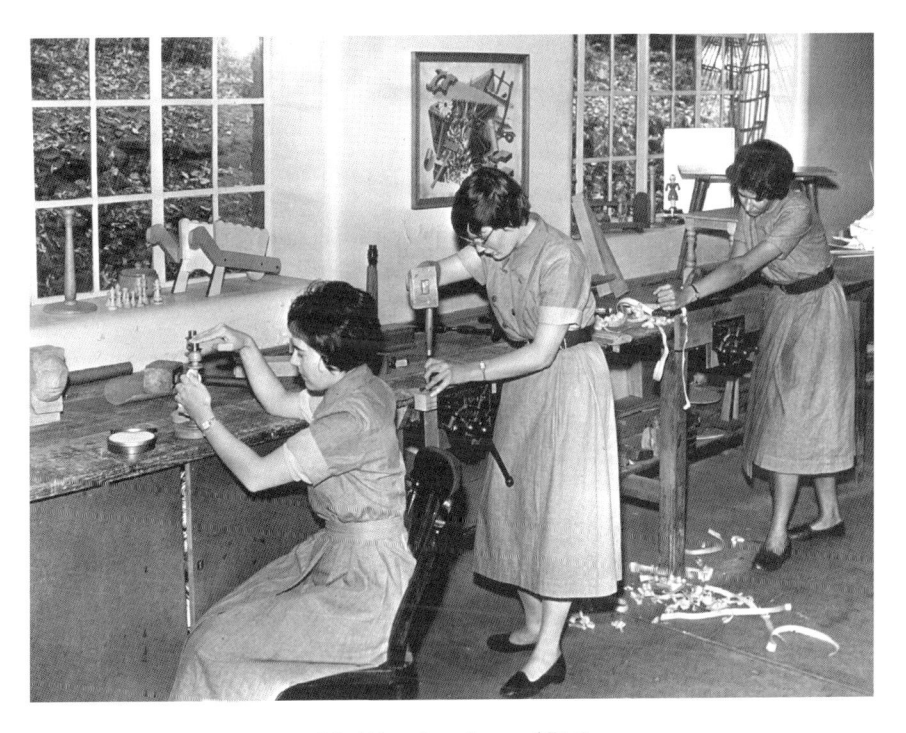

13. Woodwork ca. 1950s

Certain cafés in the town became favourite haunts – the Wedgwood on Abington Street, for instance, (still standing opposite the top of St. Giles Terrace). Here time might be whiled away drinking coffee before going to the Grand Hotel on Gold Street for lunch (now closed). However, *'the great thing was to take a bicycle down to the town and go to the Clipper'.* This was another café, in the basement of the present

Adams bakery on the corner of Wood Hill and St. Giles Street. The interior was decked out like the inside of an airliner. The students could afford to sit there all evening with one cup of coffee. The waitresses were dressed as air stewardesses, and Osborne Robinson, a local scenic designer, had painted circular scenes to resemble views through an aeroplane window. *'Saturday mornings everybody, but everybody went down to the Derngate Café* (above the former bus station on the site of the Derngate Theatre). *'This was where young people in general met to decide what they were going to do in the evening. The occupational therapists used to go down in force, and if you wanted to meet anybody, that's where you went.'*

Sometimes friends would hitchhike to London to see a show, go home overnight and then hitch a lift back again – *'at times a very close shave to make it by the late pass time of midnight'*. Of course the curfew of 10.30 pm is always well remembered – more particularly, how to get round it. To start with, only one late key was allowed per half term, later being increased to once a week, so various methods were employed to get back into the hostel without the warden noticing your absence. You might leave a rope hanging out of your room window. When pulled this would lift the lid off the linen basket and waken your two room-mates who could open the fire escape door or a downstairs window for you. A more primitive method involved throwing a pebble up at the appropriate room, or even just arranging for a downstairs window to be left open. You might have to be careful of course not to burn your legs on the solid radiators beneath the windows. Climbing over the railings was a useful feat to master, or shinning up the high wall round Rheinfelden. You may only have been late because you were babysitting, but if you had been out with a boyfriend ('a follower') you had to say good night at the end of the road. Followers were not allowed to escort you to the door, and as the warden always liked to meet them, they would be invited in one afternoon for a cup of tea.

Meeting young men did not prove difficult despite Northampton's reputation. Two past students have described how the town was said to be the most difficult place to get into socially *'because it was such an incestuous place in a way – so much inter-marriage among families that had been here for generations.'* *'It was like no other town in England because it was so completely self-contained, almost in the middle of the country, and it hadn't changed for hundreds of years ... It did have a very special ambience about it – a very interesting place.'* Mrs. Hombersley encouraged her students to go to different churches in order to meet people. The Young Farmers group was also suggested as a suitable social venue. The Saturday dances at the Art College were popular, although the room was very small and students were crammed in until there was literally no room to move. More pleasant were the occasional dances which the students organised themselves in the upstairs room at the Wedgwood.

Cycling was evidently an important form of transport, with almost everyone having a bike in the 1940s. Students doing a placement at the

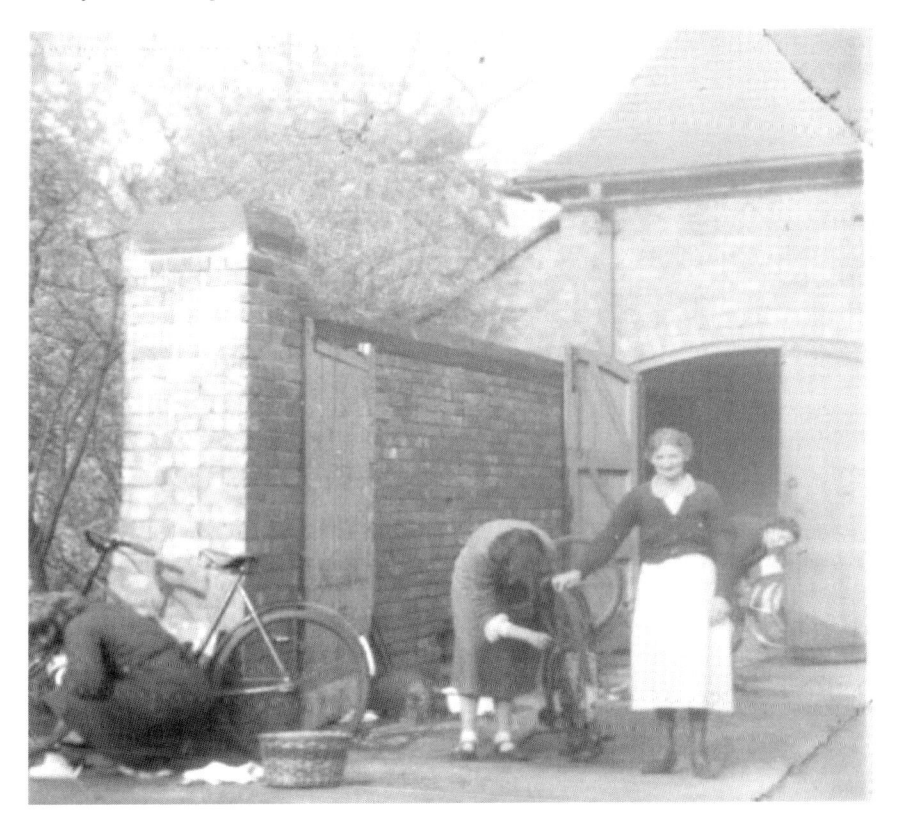

14. Repairing bicycles 1950s

Creaton Sanatorium were even prepared to cycle the ten miles out to this village set in the pretty hilly countryside north of the town. Some students also used their bicycles to explore at weekends or even to have a trip to Stratford and Cambridge, about 40 miles away from Northampton. *'Every Saturday and Sunday (if we were not on duty somewhere) we went off with a picnic to see a church. In those days they were all open and we read the inscriptions on some extraordinary tombs ... We also used to cycle over to Stratford, book into a small hotel, sit on a small stool in the gallery to see the afternoon performance, grab some fish and chips and sit on a stool to see the evening performance. Then we'd stay and cycle home the next day. I know my mother had the police out looking for us once. We'd cycled to Cambridge to see my friend's brother and stayed at the YWCA. My mother knew when we were due back the next day, but it was so difficult. It was VE night and I had a puncture on the way home. We saw this house with lights on and knocked on the back door to see if they could help. There was a chauffeur there and a party on. They were celebrating. They were so kind to us. The chauffeur fixed my puncture and they gave us sandwiches and milk and we set off again. We got to Northampton in about an hour, although the wretched tyre went down again. The police were out looking for us. I think we got home about 1 o'clock.'* Closer to home fine summer days saw the students swimming in the outdoor pool at Midsummer Meadow, just down the hill from the hostel. The more adventurous ones even swam nearby in the locks in the river at Becket's Park.

The exhuberant energy of the students inevitably expressed itself in the tricks they got up to. The front lawns at St. Andrew's were strictly out of bounds; in the dark the girls would dare each other to cross them. Nicknamed 'the sacred turf' the lawns were the ideal setting to install the skeleton from the lecture theatre, dressed in a student uniform and scarf, or draped on a chair like a drunk, a champagne bottle in his hand. Dr. Tennent and Mrs. Hombersley were not amused. The students were also said to be not averse to letting the tyres down on the bicycle of a young doctor who came to lecture them on anatomy. However, the initiation ceremony that is remembered from the early 50s was something that got out of hand and was eventually banned. *'The first years were invited to a party in the lounge of Rheinfelden and were taken singly, blindfolded outside to the old coach house at the back and up the stairs to the loft, where they were made to kneel in front of a low table. They had to bow to St. Andrew three times, each time touching the table with their forehead. The third time a bowl of water was pushed forward so their head went in. They were given a towel to dry themselves with, but it was well lathered with flour.'*

Some of the students managed to fit in time for a job alongside their academic and practical work. Babysitting was a favourite, and there was a steady demand from local families and members of staff at the hospital. Working on the hospital switchboard was another convenient option. Some jobs required the permission of Mrs. Hombersley, such as working as a cinema usherette. Where the environment was not considered safe or salubrious, a taxi would be organised to bring the student back to her hostel: *'Pauline worked as a waitress in a rather* doubtful café in Bridge Street. Bridge Street was doubtful then – full of American airmen. She was strictly escorted there and back.' St. Andrew's offered voluntary work with free board and lodging at their Welsh holiday home, Bryn-y-Neuadd. 'It was a nice holiday job. One of the many activities we engaged in was to accompany (some hundred yards behind) a rather wild and energetic lady who liked climbing mountains!'

Social life was punctuated by two major events in the School's calendar – the St. Andrew's Night ball and the Garden Party. The ball seems to be etched in the memory of all the students from this time. It began in 1946 and was the brainchild of Mrs. Hombersley who gave two of her local students a challenge that tested their social skills and diplomacy in true occupational therapy fashion. 'Mrs. H. had a bright idea ... She said to Rosemary Bull and me, "I think we should have a ball and I want you two to find 50 young men". Our local girlfriends were not a bit pleased about it, and so I said to Mrs. H., "Look, if there are two boys in one family and a sister, am I just to ask the boys? – because I can't do it." And she said, "Oh very well, you can ask the sister". I knew that one of my friends wouldn't let me invite her boyfriend – "You're not having John!" ' The names of the boys all went into what became known as the Eligibles Book. 'Quite apart from the young eligibles, if we were going to invite any young men as escorts to the ball we had to have written approval from our parents.' Most of the eligibles were the sons of wealthy shoe manufacturers, but it became the goal of many a young man to get on the list. One young PhD graduate achieved success: 'We heard about this list and thought "We've got to get on it somehow". So my friend wrote a letter saying he was new to the area and all that and signed it "Dr. John Wood". He'd studied physics, but of course Mrs. H. thought he was a medical doctor. Once he got on, well, myself and two or three others got on too.' The Book was passed down from year to year, each year crossing out names which seemed to have been there too long.

The food on these occasions was magnificent – glazed pig's head and all, but there was no alcohol. Needless to say, smuggling in bottles of drink in cars proved one way round the ban. The dress code and standards of behaviour were very strict, formal replies being expected. 'Mrs. H. remonstrated with my boyfriend (for not replying) and he said he was terribly sorry but at Cambridge they just didn't do this. Of course he charmed her.' The resourceful students would set to making their own dresses and even the gloves to match. Some chose such full-skirted styles that the task of hemming the yards and yards of material proved too much, one girl deciding to go to the ball with her skirt neatly pinned instead. Even the cost of material could be excessive and the bargains on the market were very appealing. However, in the refined atmosphere of the School there seemed to be such a stigma attached to buying off the market that one student pretended she'd bought hers in the local department store: *'I was busily constructing my dress one evening when Mrs. H. came in. 'What are you doing?' So I explained and she said "That's nice material; where did you get it?" I thought if I tell her I got it off the market, she'll think me dreadful, so I said I bought it in Adnitt's. "Oh", she said, "You don't want to waste your money in there. You want to go to the market!"* '

A few trustworthy patients might be invited to the ball. *'I remember one such: tall, handsome and immaculate in tails and white gloves, but with the disconcerting habit of wandering into the middle of the Great Hall between dances to pick up threads or something that only he could see, and then he'd blow them from his fingertips. We were told not to reveal to 'outsiders' that some patients were attending the ball.'*

The Garden Party coincided with the graduation ceremony and Open Day. For the students it meant a new dress and a new hat. The afternoon began with a service in the chapel, presided over by an eminent local personage. The Bishop of Peterborough once gave the sermon. This was followed by the second years' exhibition of work, tea in the garden of Priory Cottage and the presentation of prizes. By 1953 the number of graduates attending was growing and the decision was taken to form a Graduates' Association. By 1954 a committee had adopted a constitution and made plans for a weekend conference in November where papers were to be read, a talk given on the new syllabus, and a demonstration of paper sculpture. (Sadly the Graduates' Association declined in subsequent years and ceased to exist.)

The social life and grand social occasions of the students provide an insight into the unfamiliar post-war world of the late 1940s and early 50s – an important background to the early development of the School. The syllabus itself was quite hard, but one of the lighter sides of the curriculum was Physical Recreation. It had always been an important part of occupational therapy at St. Andrew's. Girls would be asked to take patients swimming at the municipal baths on Saturday mornings or give tennis coaching, for example. There were seven grass courts on the area between the chapel and the golf course – the best grass courts for miles and the home ground of the County tennis team. Every year there used to be an inter-hospital tennis match involving the General Hospital, St. Andrew's and St. Crispin's, among others. It took place at St. Crispin's and the huge silver cup for which they played was placed on display. *'The cup was placed on a chair by the side of the court. Halfway through the* match we'd go and have tea in the hospital and the cup was just left there. Eventually they decided to have it valued and it was worth thousands of pounds. We had just left it on the chair!' Girls might even play in the hockey team. Matches had to be held in the hospital grounds in order to provide entertainment for the patients. This requirement somewhat restricted the ambitions of the students who were good

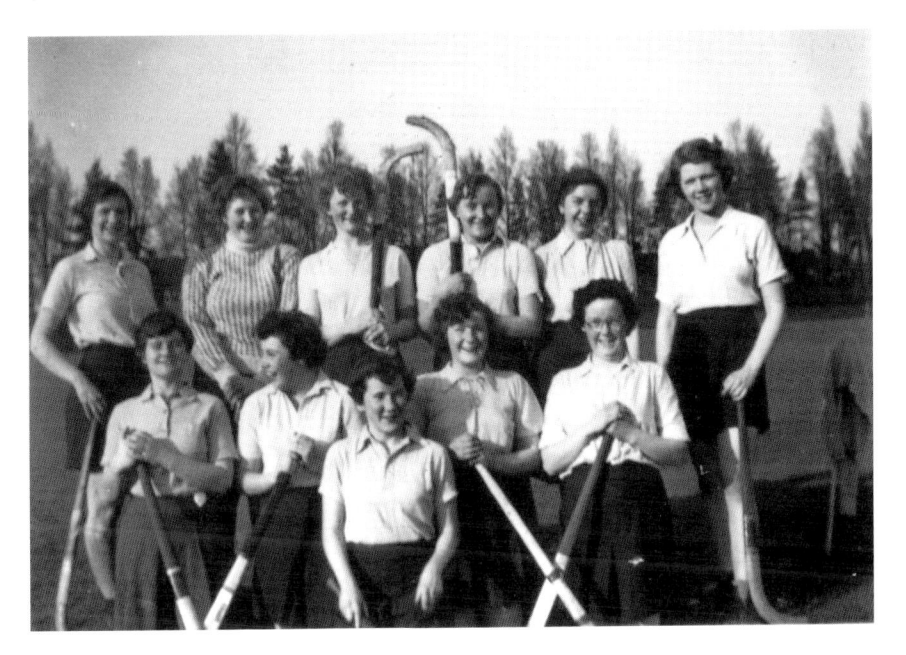

15. Hockey Team 1952

hockey players. The honour of being invited to play for the Northampton town team was short-lived, for Dr. Tennent heard about it and said 'Nonsense – we'll have a hockey team at the hospital.' 'We formed a team at St. Andrew's and they provided us with a bright red and green uniform. Mrs. Tennent played and some doctors and a few nurses. We were lethal, but we did pretty well. Dr. Tennent wouldn't let us go out to play because we had to entertain the patients.' A more active participation by the patients took place on the annual Sports Day which seems to have re-started in 1954. Dr. Tennent was pleased that by far the greater proportion of the participants were patients.

Mrs. Latto, from the Central Council for Physical Recreation, was employed in 1948 in order to teach the students PE, which they did clad in grey pleated shorts and a white blouse. She also taught other activities which could be used with the patients, such as national and country dancing, and the students had to plan a programme of taught activities for a whole term. They worked with the patients in the lessons, encountering some hazards along the way. 'You had to choose a partner to dance with. My partner was known to be quite manic at times. She was a woman and she had her hand in the middle of my back. I could feel her hand getting tighter and tighter as we waltzed round. The music then stopped but we didn't, and in the end she ripped my shirt right across from one end to the other. We landed in a heap on the dance floor. The patient was taken back to the ward – music had that effect on her. It was a good lesson; you had to know who it was you'd got in your group.'

Physical recreation was linked with all the various social events which were laid on for the patients and in which the students were expected to take part. The events provided further useful experience in organisation and management. It is thought that the first play to be produced in the hospital was 'The Bishop's Candlesticks' in 1945 – produced by Mrs. Tennent and acted in by several of the students. When Mrs. Hombersley arrived she decided to make a Christmas pantomime an annual event to be arranged by the students themselves. She produced the first one in 1948 – 'Snow White and the Seven Dwarves', and thereafter the girls were on their own. The production of '1066 and All That' in the early 50s is particularly remembered for the scene in which a group of students danced the can-can and then proceeded down the steps to the audience to sit on the laps of those in the front-row, including Dr. Tennent.

By 1955 the patients were being encouraged to participate in the Christmas entertainment, even if it was behind the scenes making costumes, scenery and props. Regular play readings became so popular that they had to be limited to 'members', chosen as being those patients who would derive the maximum therapeutic benefit. 1958 saw the most ambitious play yet – 'Aladdin', which was a joint effort again by patients, staff and students, and even involved the patients in writing parts of the script.

Once a month a dance was held for the patients, and once a week two of the students were responsible for organising a social with games and other activities. The ballroom dancing classes for students and patients, which started in 1950, provided a useful basis for the monthly dances. One student recalls taking patients on outings to Stratford and London, and although this was when she was no longer a student, it is an interesting reflection of the relaxed attitude to safety in those days. Patients might be taken to the theatres or exhibitions. 'We never really had any trouble. We never lost a patient. We jolly nearly lost one. There was a big funfair and one girl decided to go for a ride on one of the big wheels. Fortunately, she'd got both legs in plaster so she couldn't walk very fast. When we got back to the coach, I said, "There's one missing". Of course it was rather difficult to find her but we saw these legs sticking out on the big wheel. So we got her back ... The patients were lovely. I don't know how mad they were. They all had their sort of dignity.' Alongside the various social events which brought the students in contact with the patients, the girls were encouraged to read the newspapers in order to be able to converse with them. Not only were the patients' social skills being developed, the students were also learning to improve their art of conversation.

Despite the development of the students' relationship with the patients, a certain distance had to be maintained. Christian names, for example, were not to be used despite some patients' eager efforts at discovery. Near disasters happened when the students were still inexperienced on the wards. 'I remember the first time I went along to a locked ward, somebody said to me, "Oh I've forgotten my lighter. Could you let me out?" And I did, and then I thought I shouldn't have done that. I rushed along to Dr. O'Connell's office and said I thought I'd done something wrong because I'd let a patient out who'd gone to get his lighter. So he went flying off ... I suppose the patient was going to set fire to something. He was an arsonist.'

Although it might seem to put a certain pressure on the staff and students, daily visits to the wards by Dr. Tennent or Dr. O'Connell were often welcomed. 'It was wonderful to know that you might have a visit ... Later when I went to work and never saw the medical superintendent I really got rather down about it.'

As St. Andrew's was a private hospital, some of the patients were famous people. The students soon learned to be souls of discretion and not to reveal who it was they were helping to treat. Sometimes they have recalled with affection the behaviour of particular patients with whom they came into contact. Phyllis Castle in her book, 'Memoirs of a Misfit', includes a particularly entertaining story of one of her St. Crispin's patients who suffered from delusions of grandeur.

'It wasn't until I went on outside clinical practice in the local mental hospital that I met my favourite character. He wasn't in my class, but kept trying to gate-crash, only to find himself blocked by the charge nurse, a huge, white-coated fellow with the figure of a base-line rugby football player. The patient was small and lightly built, it didn't seem fair. True, he thought of himself as Napoleon Bonaparte, but that was not his appearance. He looked like an addled Eliot. As soon as I saw him I *noticed the resemblance to the poet. In fact, he was a native of the Channel Islands, who'd worked for some years in France. But none of this tied in with his hair – plastered forward and licked back with a pinch at the front, twiddled up to an uncertain point on top of his head.*

"But I want to do some knitting, sir, the lady said I could." He wasn't well enough behaved, I was told. But he persisted, and, in the end, he got his way.

"What's he making, is it a vest?" asked the big man. It was undeniably a curious shape with gaping holes. He was always delighted to be put right and then forged vigorously ahead with his own variations as before. When I told him it was 'individual', he was tickled. "Is it? Looks fine to me. Just the thing for the car! When I finish this I'll be doing one for the wife." He was always enchanting to listen to. When the going was strong, he owned the hospital, Selfridge's and the Marble Arch. "I've been given a Rolls. An exceedingly large lump sum has been settled on me". With millions coming in each day it was nothing to him. "I've written to the Bank of England", I was assured as he tore off a piece of newsprint, carefully folded it down to size and slotted it into the hospital mail box. Straight out of the text-book into real life – 'delusions of grandeur' in person!

'Somehow I managed to get him off the terrible knitting, onto a rug in herringbone stitch. He got on better with this – could even see when he went wrong and was pleased by the green areas in the pattern. "My Intelligence Corps colours!" Fact or fancy? And when I spoke of the design as 'symmetrical', he at once picked up the word and dandled it. All the same I couldn't help feeling mean, he really loved that unbelievable knitting. The dilemma was resolved when he was given permission to do a short session every evening before going to bed.

'Unlike the rest of the class, there was hope for the addled Eliot. He'd been put on a stringent new heat treatment, and if his body could tolerate this long enough, it should have been only a question of time. Splendidly, classically deranged as he was, he'd been able to take this on board, he knew he'd been seriously ill, but should now get better. And this mixed situation was reflected in his behaviour – sensible enough, at other times clearly enclosed in a flamboyant world of his own.

'He was already looking less addled. "I talk too much", he said of himself, "I must get on with my work" We reached the stage where he saw that the others put their things away tidily at the end of the morning, he then ran round putting the room to rights. "They are funny, aren't they?" he said of the class. But I didn't find them funny. I couldn't get through to them. I put their work right and that was it.

'Then came the morning that changed everything. I arrived to find him waiting for me at the hospital entrance. "Miss! – at two o'clock this morning my mind came back! Yes, I'm all right now." And he was – he

remembered his past, he knew who he was, and all that stuff about elephants, yachts and cars was only because he'd been ill. The trouble had been general paralysis of the insane, G.P.I., a late manifestation of syphilis that usually appears eight to twenty years after infection, causing fearful havoc in both body and mind.

'But syphilis, I soon discovered, was more than just one disease, it was an Empire – a marshalling of sophisticated bacterial organisms – agile, thread-like presences with a taste for whizzing round in the most vital parts of their host. They also had a talent for acting under cover, imitating other infectious diseases, TB and leprosy for preference. But this time they'd been outmanoeuvred – this particular late-flowering performance had led to extinction.

'By the time my clinical practice in the hospital finished, he was going home every weekend. He was picking up but still looked under strain. He'd been admitted sick – a triumphant Napoleon. He was going out cured – as it appeared – sad and defeated. The hospital had saved his life. He had now to prove himself.'

Phyllis' overall personal reaction to her work with psychiatric patients was a sense of being imprisoned, oppressed by the maintenance of restraint, and the need for caution hanging heavy in the air. She admits to being unaware of her reaction at the time, but recalls the feeling of relief she experienced on starting work in a physical hospital. *'And then it hit me. It was so unexpected it came as a shock. People were <u>communicating</u> with each other. They were making jokes, laughing, pulling legs ... The first half of our training (at St. Andrew's) amounted to a virtual immersion in the mental side of our work ... That I'd been so totally unaware was what alarmed me.'* So the students reacted in different ways to the psychiatric training, some seeking a return to more normal ways of social interaction and others relishing the challenges it presented.

In the mid 1950s some of the students have less fond memories of the grandeur and dignity of life at St. Andrew's. It seems amazing now, but the third years, after their finals, had two weeks before they could go home because their parents had paid for a term of a certain length and they were to be given their money's worth. Each student had to spend one day of that two weeks working in the hospital laundry. The experience was supposed to be educational, for all large psychiatric hospitals employed their patients in this way. *'They had to find something for us to do. They sent us to work in the laundry. It was the hottest day of the year – in the 80s and 90s. There we were in our uniforms done up*

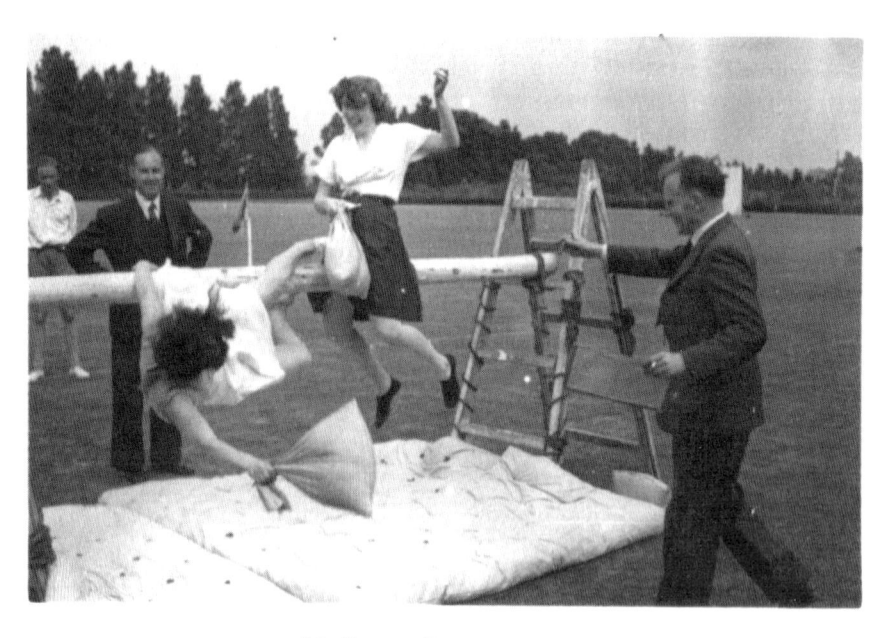

16. Sports Day ca. 1950s

to the neck. I have never been so hot in my life, or felt so miserable. I think working in the hospital laundry in the mid 1950s was the worst thing anybody could have asked us to do. It was stinking. It was filthy. We were put on to do the bed-sheets when they came out of the boiling coppers. They were put on an enormous steam-fed roller which was the width of a sheet, and you fed the sheet on and it rolled round. The roller was just pumping out dry steam heat the whole time. You had to be careful not to burn your hand or get it caught in the rollers.'

Overall Mrs. Hombersley felt justly proud of her students. The School had grown immediately after the war and then maintained a steady intake of about twenty students per year. Exam results had fluctuated, but in 1957 they were found to be very good – 90% had passed the Diploma, with 71 credits and 76 distinctions in individual exams. There had always been individual students who had attained particularly good marks – in 1956 for the second time a St. Andrew's student won the A.O.T. prize for the highest marks in the Diploma exams. In reporting on the results of 1957 Dr. Tennent quite rightly pointed out that it was a reflection of the dedication of the various tutors. In actual fact some of the lecturers are remembered more for their eccentricities than their teaching, but others clearly made a special impression on the students. *'One psychiatrist was as mad as a hatter ... He paced all the time when he was lecturing us, and every now and then he'd do a sort of run at the wall ... He had a blackboard on an easel. He'd be lecturing on some aspect of psychology and would be writing on the blackboard. He'd come to the edge of the board, hadn't finished his sentence, so he'd go on round the back.'*

Neville Parsons-Jones is remembered with great affection. Born in 1920, he had joined St. Andrew's staff in 1934 and retired in 1978 after 44 years. He was a registered mental nurse before becoming an occupational therapist in 1949, in 1954 taking study leave to complete the dual qualification and obtain a full Diploma. In 1967 he became Head of the Department. *'His caring, creative and positive approach to treatment laid the foundation stones for the development and respect of the profession and department at the hospital ... PJ guided and taught many of today's practising occupational therapists. A gentle and compassionate man, he always had time to listen to his patients and colleagues, and continued to care for his staff and patients after his retirement.'* So runs his obituary in the staff magazine after his death in 1989. Some of his students from the 1950s have shared their memories of his character and kindness: *'He was an amazing teacher, so easy to get on with. He had a workshop full of male patients and of course these patients were often mucking around. He was quite a strict man. He must have been in the medical services in the army during the war and was made a PoW. Out of one of his cupboards he produced a little bowl made of strips of paper that he'd made when a PoW. The strips were 6" long and about ¾" wide and had been rolled into a tube. They were stuck together to make a little bowl. The PoWs used to keep their scraps of paper and make glue paste out of bread and water. Not many of the bowls survived. The mice liked to eat them.'* ... *'I was making a coffee table and was trying to saw the legs – they were to be made from a plank of cedar. I'd gone to the canteen for a coffee and when I came back, PJ had sawn it all for me and put it back together like a jigsaw. I suppose he realised there's a limit to how much an 18 year old arm can cope with. He very kindly had finished the sawing for me. He was a lovely man.'*

Elin Dallas arrived at the School in 1953 and took over from Miss Stamper as Deputy Director of Training. Much of the drama work with the patients, which has been described on previous pages, took place thanks to Miss Dallas' arrival. Her story belongs in the next chapter for she went on to take over from Mrs. Hombersley in 1957. It must however be said that along with PJ, she played an important part in providing the broad colourful course which the students were able to follow.

The last words on this period in the School's history should go to Mrs. Hombersley. They are taken from a speech she made to doctors in 1952, based partly on her acute awareness of the needs and opportunities of the occupational therapy profession: '*After some years of experiment I have come to the conclusion that one cannot teach Occupational Therapy. One can indicate fundamentals in lectures, but the student has got to learn the hard way – by trying herself. No one can do this for her and the most we, as teachers, can do for her is to give her a good example and tell her when she is going wrong. If we have selected wisely she will learn from her own mistakes and will continue to learn throughout her professional career. Much of her value to you will depend on this willingness to learn and experiment.*

'*Dr. FitzGerald has mentioned some of the qualities of personality which he hopes an Occupational Therapist will possess. All her training and in particular her clinical experience is designed to develop her personality. The student will have acquired certain manual skills in the treatment of her patients. She will also have learnt that she needs more than her craftwork in the exercise of her profession. She will be prepared to use anything which comes to hand as a therapeutic aid – whether this is the shelling of peas or the stripping of blackcurrants – the doing of a crossword puzzle – the selection of suitable reading matter for her patients from the hospital library – production of a pantomime for the patients – the organisation of a gramophone recital – physical training in all its aspects, from a simple exercise class to a square dance session or a tennis tournament.*

'*She will have learnt gradually to accept responsibility at first for her own actions – then for a small group of patients until finally she can carry willingly and without strain the responsibility which will be hers when she starts to practise her profession as a fully qualified individual. I hope that by the time our rather raw, ill balanced but enthusiastic 18 year old reaches this stage she will have retained her enthusiasm but will be able to temper it with good judgement – that she will have learnt the self-control which is necessary before one can control others – that she will have grown in sympathy and understanding of her patient's needs and will be equipped to supply those needs – that she will be observant and will have learned how to express herself clearly and concisely both on paper and in words – and above all that she will have learnt to put herself in the other person's place, whether that person is a patient or a member of staff. Only so will she be able to maintain that good relationship which is the foundation of any successful work ...*

'We are a new profession and the recognition you have given us devoting a session to the discussion of our problems is a great encouragement. We are doing our best to give you good Occupational Therapists. We are very conscious of their shortcomings and know how much they still have to learn. I am confident, however, that under your wise guidance they will develop into really helpful members of your treatment team.'

Chapter 4

Signs of Change

Elin Dallas 1957 – 1972

Swinging Sixties – Students in general start to object to rules while away studying – 1962 Education Act gives mandatory grants to all Higher Education students – Onset of rising inflation - Move to give more independence to disabled people – Rise in number of people with learning disabilities, elderly with senile dementia, and people with traumatic brain injuries – 1959 Mental Health Act encourages care in the community.
Image of occupational therapy becomes less certain in 1960s – Watershed decade for the profession as focus shifts to ADL – 1966 C.O.T. begins new four yearly inspections of Schools.

The sense of the newness of the profession, so evident in Joyce Hombersley's talk, might explain why the image of occupational therapy was so fragile and uncertain in the 1960s. In this decade dramatic changes took place in medicine and social policy and the profession could perhaps be said to lose its footing. The 1960s has in fact been described as a watershed decade for the profession – a time when the focus very definitely shifted to the physical aspect of providing aids for disabled people. These changes could create a few problems for the training schools as they sought to keep up with the new demands made upon them.

Elin Dallas arrived at Northampton in 1953 and took over from Mrs. Hombersley on her retirement in 1957, remaining at the School until 1973. Born in London in 1908, she trained as a classical Greek dancer and had been on tour in Europe. She subsequently trained at the Dorset House School of Occupational Therapy; she may even have been taught by Elizabeth Casson herself and was influenced and inspired by the revolutionary sense of creativity which lay behind so much of Casson's ideas. Before coming to Northampton Miss Dallas had been in charge of the Occupational Therapy department at Birmingham Children's Hospital, a place where her love of creativity would have had much practical value among the young patients.

One of her students has suggested that Miss Dallas brought Elizabeth Casson's pioneering spirit to the St. Andrew's School. *'It was a very young profession (and yet we felt it had been going forever). Now I look back and think it was in its infancy. Pioneers like Elizabeth Casson were having an influence on it because they taught future teachers like Miss Dallas. She didn't quote Elizabeth Casson a lot but she must have been using those techniques. No wonder she did a lot of dance. We were very much part of the pioneers. Now people I work with regard me as a pioneer, which seems strange. They talk to me almost as if I was one of the originals.'*

Combined with her creativity was an eccentricity which did not help in her administrative role. Although the School grew and generally flourished during the fifteen years Miss Dallas was Principal, in the mid 60s various problems became evident which will be described in the course of this chapter. First of all, however, the School's development must be set in the context of the dramatic changes in medicine and social policy mentioned earlier.

In 1959 the Mental Health Act introduced changes in the treatment of the mentally ill that led the Medical Director of St. Andrew's in 1974 to claim that psychiatric hospitals had changed more in the past twenty years than in the previous hundred. One of the main principles behind the Act was the reorientation of mental health services away from institutional care towards care in the community. This new attitude must be seen in the light of the facts that by the mid 1950s mental hospitals and homes for people with learning disabilities were seriously overcrowded, and there was an acute shortage of psychiatric nursing and junior medical staff. Mental illness was to be treated in the same way as physical illness, so patients could enter a mental hospital on the same basis as they would a nursing home or general hospital. Admission would now be much more informal without the need for a patient to be 'sectioned' by a magistrate using his powers of detention. Compulsory admission was still possible, but safeguards were put in place so that patients had the right of appeal.

The number of long stay patients in places like St. Andrew's declined rapidly therefore. By 1969 there were 20% fewer than in the 1950s. The Medical Director, Dr. Harper, suggested this was the most significant development in the whole range of medicine since the conquest of tuberculosis as an epidemic disease in the years immediately after the Second World War. However, regarding the growing need for occupational therapy, it is important to note his subsequent comments on how the number of people with learning disabilities or elderly people suffering from senile dementia was on the increase, as more of the former were reaching adulthood and as people lived longer. He also pointed out the rise in the number of people who survived road accidents, leading to a greater number of physically disabled and brain injured people. All these client groups are people who are treated by occupational therapists.

The demands therefore made on occupational therapists in the context of a mental hospital began to change. Their 'diversional' work with long stay residents reduced as more were prepared for life back in the community. Also, in the field of physical disability changes were taking place that had a similar effect on the type of treatment which could be offered. There was a move to enable greater independence among physically disabled people, partly as a result of the new ethos on their rights as individuals, and partly because advances in medicine were reducing the length of time spent in hospital and hence the time spent on extensive rehabilitation programmes. Discharge from hospital had to be carefully planned so that domestic tasks did not present a problem when the patient went home. One of the students remembers the huge weaving looms at Manfield Orthopaedic Hospital used to rehabilitate the patients with various joint injuries in the 1950s, and how by 1971 they were no longer in use. Nowadays in the 21st century knee operations can be performed by keyhole surgery for which a patient need not even stay overnight. So the innovative adaptation of equipment to rehabilitate a patient's injured limb gradually became a less important occupational therapy skill.

These changes in the treatment of mental illness and physical injury meant that the assessment of patients prior to discharge into the community and/or their home became very important. It was a task that fell naturally to occupational therapists, but one which had not previously featured to any great extent in their training in the 1940s and 50s. To be of value, assessment needed to be scientific in its precision, and calls were made for the diploma to be upgraded to a degree to ensure a higher status for the profession. Occupational therapists had to be able to identify their patient's medical state and social performance, as well as his/her ability to work. The time required for accurate assessment was found sometimes to be longer than the time that might have been taken for treatment.

One thing had not changed. There was still an acute shortage of occupational therapists. Membership of the A.O.T. was up to 2358 in 1960, but there were no fewer than 655 vacant posts. The A.O.T. could see how occupational therapy had expanded and diversified, so the committee called for a clear restatement of the aims and functions of the profession. They also drew attention to the need for a closer liaison with all allied workers, such as physiotherapists and social workers – an aspect of work which was a relatively new concept at the time but is now the norm; 'networking' is a familiar term in many professions now. The fear for the future of occupational therapy surfaced again, although couched in different terms from those expressed by Joyce Hombersley in the early 1950s. Rita Goble, a prominent spokeswoman, declared that occupational therapy was *'not so much a profession at the moment as a group of technocrats operating within medicine.'*

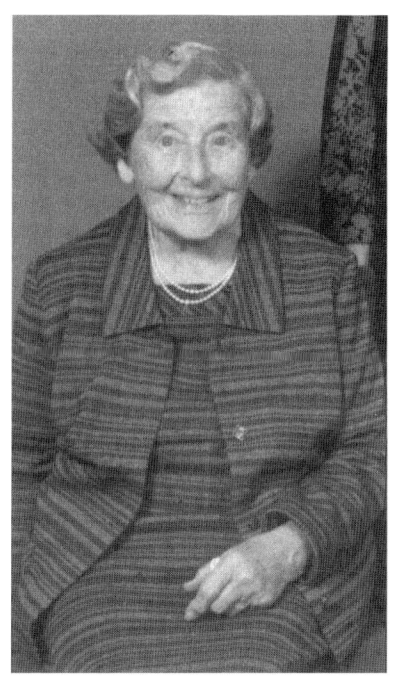

17. *Elin Dallas*

When Miss Dallas took over the School in 1957 she seemed to have little idea of the difficulties ahead. Students have varying attitudes towards her. Some remember her as *'a character – the exact opposite of Mrs. Hombersley – not very strict'*. *'You didn't have much difficulty in pulling the wool over her eyes. She didn't tell people off very much.'* Yet she is also described as *'very commanding, very frightening in her own way'*. She had an upsetting tendency to treat her students' craftwork as her own. *'She'd say, "I'll give that as a leaving present for one of the doctors", and you'd have spent absolutely days on it. She just said, "Yes, darling, go and make another rug".'* Others simply remember her as an eccentric – *'mad, quite, quite mad'*. During her time as Principal there were several foreign students, from Nigeria and Sweden for example. She kept a fond eye on their well-being and is remembered with affection by at least one of them – one of the Nigerians still appreciating her concern for his welfare. She is also remembered for the care which she took in obtaining the right clinical practice for a particular student. *'She had very grand ideas about her students and sometimes she was very, very good. She really did try to get the right hospital practice for you. I remember she tried to match the right placement to the right student.'*

She obviously had a way with the patients and got on well with them, being involved as Head of Department as well as Director of Training: *'I remember once we were out in the grounds taking some patients for a walk, and we'd got this elderly lady wrapped up in an enormous fur coat. It was the height of summer and she was absolutely sweltering, so we thought we'd better get her back to the ward, but she'd got a phobia about turning left. So we were just going round and round in circles. We sent one of the others off to find Miss Dallas to come and help us. She came along, took the lady by the arm and said, "Why are you making all this fuss? You know your way back to the ward." And off she took her. She obviously had a knack with the patients.'*

Miss Dallas lived in a cottage at Moulton Park on land owned by St. Andrew's. (The farm here was a source of occupation for some of the male patients but was closed in 1962, work then being provided in the gardens. The villa on the farm, used as a residence for some female patients, remained open.) Later on Miss Dallas shared the cottage with her new deputy, Maria Van Garderen. For whoever lived or worked with her, it did not take long to discover that Miss Dallas was devoted to her cats. Even at interviews with prospective students the cats she kept at the School were in evidence, sometimes pawing at the interview papers. One student came all the way from Ireland to attend for interview on the School's Open Day. The first words Miss Dallas spoke to her were: *'I don't know what I'm going to do. I hope it doesn't rain because the cat's wee'd on my umbrella.'* There were two girls applying from Ireland at the time and Miss Dallas had kindly offered to interview just one to save them money. At the end of the interview Imelda recalls her saying, *' "Yes, that's fine. I think you'll do. Oh, what's your friend like, by the way?" I said, "She talks more than me and she does like cats." Based on that I was accepted.'*

The interviews were not of course always as simple as that. Some students remember being asked what their father did for a living, and although it seemed a fairly normal question at the time, they look back with hindsight in horror. *'The thing that I do remember: I was asked, "What does your father do?" which was appalling. It's terrible, but that was in the days when those things were important.'* Others were more rebellious and claim to have seen a snobbish side to their Principal; *'Miss Dallas was such a snob ... We were the first to be a bit more 'grammar school' – ready to get on with being an occupational therapist rather than it was something Mummy said would be nice to do – a little bit of craft and things. I don't think she (Miss Dallas) took that very well.'* At least one girl remembers being careful how she described her father's occupation: *'He was a factory worker, but I wouldn't have got a place if I'd said that, so I said he was an electrical engineer. I can remember lying at that stage because it was really important what your parents did.'*

As the Swinging Sixties unfolded, perhaps more and more of the students resented the atmosphere of the School: *'I was educated by nuns from 5 to 17 and they were a dream compared with this place. It was so ridiculously boarding school-ish and strict and silly. I'd had a year in the art school in between, and got used to being responsible for what I did and getting on with it, and I really really enjoyed that. I went to St. Andrew's and I thought it so ridiculously strict. You had to wear the uniform the whole time, whether you were doing any hospital work or not.'*

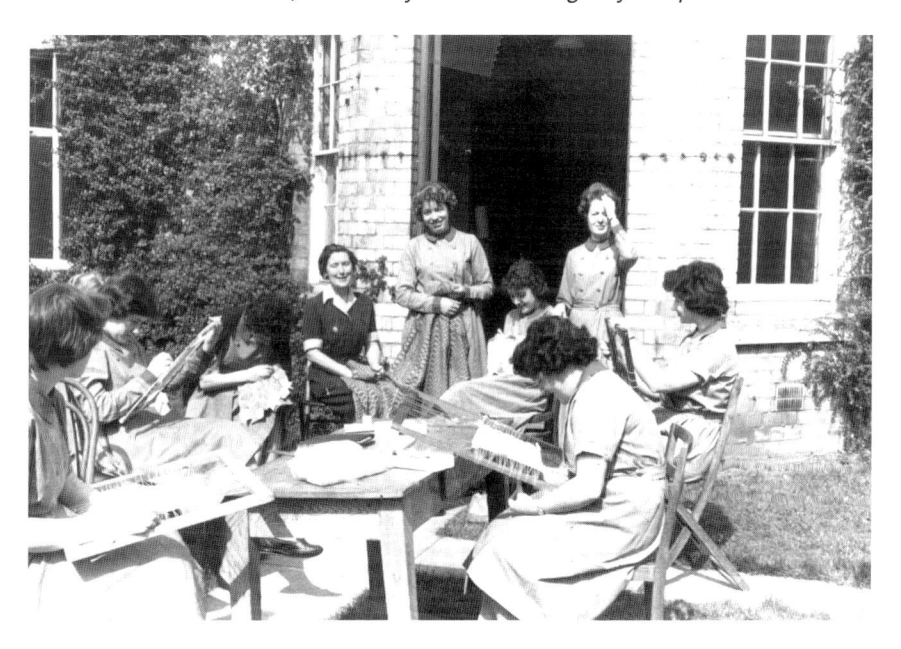

18. Embroidery class with Miss Dallas (sitting in black) 1958

The strictness also involved forbidding the students to talk to the Spanish male nurses and waiters who were being recruited in large numbers at the time. *'It was the same on clinical practice. We weren't supposed to speak to them. Occupational therapists must not speak to Spanish nurses. We were 18 to 21 but we couldn't choose who to speak to. (Of course every year someone ran off and married one or got pregnant.)'*

Perhaps one recollection epitomises the caring yet eccentric side of Miss Dallas: *'Dilly would make us stand up for lectures for half an hour or so because she said it was good practice for ward rounds. She said, "You'll all be standing around beds when the doctor's talking to you about an orthopaedic case ... It's good for you. I'll give you a lecture now and you'll all stand up."'*

As mentioned at the beginning of this chapter, the development of the School during Miss Dallas' period as Principal reflects the nationwide changes in medicine and social policy, but they were also affected by the economic and sociological changes of the 1960s, such as the new permissiveness, the rebelliousness of young people and the onset of rising inflation, as will be seen in this and the following chapter. However, Miss Dallas' own personality and qualities also played an important role in the way in which the School changed. She was not only the Director of the School but also Head Occupational Therapist at St. Andrew's, so her love of dance and drama meant that it featured prominently in the curriculum and as an activity at the hospital. She organised the annual pantomimes, bringing together patients, staff and students. In 1958 'Aladdin' was said to be the most ambitious play yet, with patients even writing part of the script. A few years later the staging of 'Dick Whittington' created activities for the patients relating to printing, typing, painting scenery, making props, costumes and photography, apart from acting in the pantomime itself. When 'Alice in Wonderland' was staged in 1964, for the first time the work of the Assistant Stage Manager was done by one of the patients. Miss Dallas attached so much importance to the teaching of drama at the School that she would give a course of lectures on the history of drama going back to the Ancient Greeks. The dancing classes which were held included a great variety of styles ranging from Old Time, Scottish, American Square to Modern, all of which could be enjoyed at the parties held once a fortnight in the Recreation Hall. The students clearly benefited from the contact with the patients which these activities provided.

In 1960 the students were given a course on beauty culture by a qualified beautician from Atkinsons of Bond Street. A new beauty parlour was subsequently set up in the hospital which proved beneficial to the patients apart from being a novel aspect of occupational therapy. *'The patients would come in and we spent a week doing beauty therapy. We'd learn how to do a facial and hand massages, how to apply make-up and do someone's nails, and how to get the nicotine off their fingers. That was really nice. Beauty therapy and personal care were a very important part of occupational therapy.'*

In 1960 another innovation was the hospital magazine, to be run by and for the patients. Entitled 'Target', it included some excellent articles and stories on subjects ranging from Africa to Ireland to the Holy Sepulchre. Within two years it was said to be run almost entirely by the patients themselves.

The patients' art classes were another aspect of the hospital's occupational therapy activities to which the students could contribute, and in 1964 an exciting new activity was introduced – brass rubbing. Groups of up to twenty patients were taken to old churches, not only to work on the medieval brasses but to learn about the architecture and history of the building.

Physical Recreation remained an important part of the hospital's programme and students continued to be taught by Miss Latto, who came up from London once a week. One of the few students to have a car was given the task of collecting her from the railway station. The uniform had progressed now to a navy leotard with navy socks and a little navy dress on top. *'Before the days of lycra, this bright blue heavy elastic tunic, footless tights and plastic coated socks were something to behold.'* Physical Recreation involved more than just exercises. Expressive or free dance was taught, just as it had been at Dorset House under Elizabeth Casson. *'I found that very helpful, not just for work with clients later on but for my own confidence, because I think free dance is a great confidence booster. It makes you able to cope with standing up in front of somebody and making a fool of yourself.'* Sometimes ribbons and scarves were used in the dancing. The students would go to a nearby centre for children with learning disabilities where body awareness was taught. It was particularly important here, as these children have difficulty in physically avoiding people. They were encouraged to walk in time to music, moving around the other people as they did so. The combination of students learning along with patients is something which is unlikely to happen today. Miss Latto is fondly remembered as *'a very high-powered PR teacher'*.

The range of arts and crafts taught was expanding by the mid 60s to include printing, horticulture and even car maintenance, the latter being taught along with metalwork at an evening class at Delapre School. Mr. Parsons Jones reduced the amount of teaching he gave in the carpentry workshop so the beginners' level was also taught at Delapre. Although horticulture was a useful part of occupational therapy, some of the students recall how little thought had gone into the planning of the

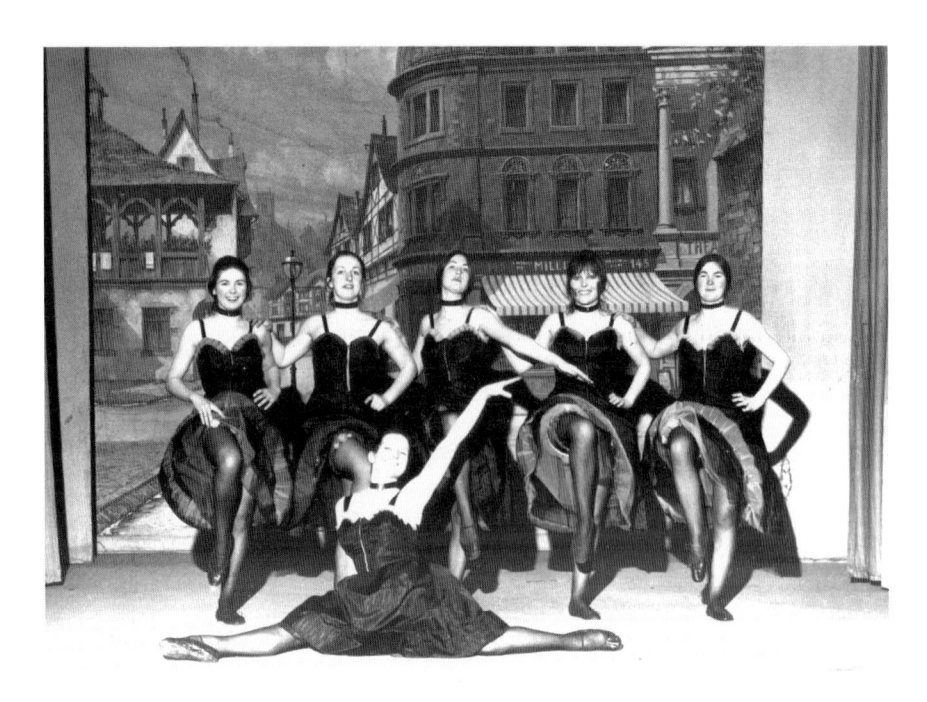

19. The Can-Can 1972

subject in the early days. '*We all turned up – about 20 or 30 of us – at the gardening hut and they would look at us and say, "What are we going to do with you all?" It could be a November morning and we'd all been told to go gardening. They used to give us a fork and rake and we'd all sweep leaves. I remember the gardening woman saying, "You're paying a lot of money to learn to be occupational therapists and all you're doing is sweeping leaves". Sometimes Dilly was not of this world almost.*'

Also by the mid 60s a new type of therapy was being introduced to St. Andrew's, thus further broadening the students' experience. Industrial workshops had been used in many psychiatric centres during the previous ten years both for rehabilitation and for the employment of patients, especially long-term ones who could not benefit from the more traditional classes. The St. Andrew's unit did work for local firms and was set up in the former billiard room. Students were given experience in creating production lines for cracker-making, for example.

Pottery was a useful craft to learn, and one which could be very therapeutic. '*We would ask the patients to do something basic like a figure representing their mother. It's amazing what would come out of that. We did use the crafts in a therapeutic way. It wasn't just for diversion.'* So important was it considered that until the School could provide its own facilities, some of the students would attend a potter's studio in the village of Brafield-on-the-Green. Here they made pots from moulds which they then decorated and fired. Numbers attending were limited, so the hospital soon tried to cater for greater numbers by providing a pottery course in the old mortuary. Here the marble slabs provided a very suitable cold surface for the clay. *'When you suddenly thought of all those dead bodies lying there in the old days, it was a bit eerie really. We did do some strange things.'* Pottery and art tutors were eventually taken on to teach the students in the evenings. By 1967 the pottery facilities on site in the hospital's occupational therapy department were being used after the patients had finished. Then in 1968 a potter's wheel was kindly donated by the Graduates Association so that the School no longer depended on using the hospital's facilities.

One final innovation that must be mentioned was the involvement of the hospital in the Northampton carnival parade. The patients prepared their float or individual entry alongside the students. Bicycles were often used, as one student well remembers. In her innocence at the time she was blissfully unaware of the meaning behind some the comments from the more rowdy onlookers. *'We all went down to Midsummer Meadow and were judged the best in our class. The funny thing was that I had a bike that was decorated with purple hearts – because at the time purple hearts were a kind of drug. I had on my cycle great big signs which said something like "I'll give you two for ten shilling". I didn't realise the double entendre. Everybody along the route was saying, "I'll give you one!"*

The academic standards of the School remained generally high, the examination results often including a good proportion of credits and distinctions. For a time some students were finding the Anatomy and Physiology course particularly difficult, but measures were taken to remedy the situation by revising the curriculum and altering the time when the subjects were examined. By 1968 a second-hand 'teaching machine' was bought for £90 to try to help the students learn these subjects. It seems to have been somewhat similar to computerised tutorials of today, being called 'programmed instruction to reinforce teaching'. Nevertheless competition among the different Schools and the advent of regular inspections by the A.O.T. and Ministry of Health meant that the School could not rely on good examination results and had to plan carefully how to balance any proposed increase in student numbers with a suitable improvement in facilities and number of staff.

In 1961 Dr. Tennent announced in his annual report that he would like to increase the intake by at least 50%, but he realised the

School would need larger premises and at present it was scattered over various rooms in the hospital. The intake went up by 25% to 25 p.a., and for the first time two male students were accepted, from Nigeria. The following year unfortunately Dr. Tennent died while on holiday in Switzerland. His former home, Priory Cottage, was a large villa in the hospital grounds and was now no longer required. It was obviously a suitable premises for the School and a fitting one also, as the School had been founded by Dr. Tennent 21 years previously. Nevertheless initially the School's move into the villa was supposed only to be temporary. There were ample classrooms and on the top floor residential accommodation for 14 students. In the same year tuition fees were increased to 240 guineas p.a. and the hostel fees to 45 guineas per term.

Some of the rooms at Priory Cottage were turned into a library and study rooms, and the external examiner's report for that year comments very favourably on the School in general: *'Students take an obvious pride in their surroundings at Priory Cottage. The School library is much in demand, and owing to improved facilities the students are able to use it for study as well as for reference.'* In 1965, as a reflection on how well established the School had now become, it is interesting to see the Medical Superintendent, Dr. O'Connell, reporting with pride on the way in which St. Andrew's School had sent out graduates to work all over the world, *'helping blind children in India, working in the only psychiatric hospital in British Guiana, finding jobs in Canada, the USA, France, Germany, Nigeria, Hong Kong and Australia.'*

The pressure for good examination results became more significant during the 60s with the advent of a new four yearly inspection of Schools by the A.O.T. and Ministry of Health, scheduled to begin in 1966. Despite the proliferation of part-time craft tutors and medical lecturers, the School still was not properly staffed. Even the Director of Training was also Head Occupational Therapist of the hospital and unable therefore to devote herself full-time to the duties of her post. Several years earlier Miss Dallas had tried to recruit a deputy but without success, probably, it is thought, because the post-holder was also required to work in the hospital. (This would rule out any applicants who were only familiar with the physical side.) Early in 1966 Miss Dallas asked to be allowed to concentrate on her role at the School and that a new Head of Department be appointed. This request was coupled with a telling letter to the Board by Mr. Parsons Jones, who subsequently accepted promotion to the post of Head. His warnings about staffing difficulties revealed the problems inherent in St. Andrew's policy of using the students as staff in the department. First of all he pointed out how he himself would not be able to fulfil the role of Head if he continued to lecture and teach practical subjects. More staff would therefore be needed. He said that the department needed an adequate and reliable number of students to help in the recreational and occupational programmes, and implied that this was not the case now: *'Ideally students should be seconded to the hospital for a period of not less than three months uninterrupted clinical practice throughout the year, as this would mean a continuity of support between resident patients, students and nursing staff.'* Occupational therapy at the hospital could even be expanded if both first and third year students were involved.

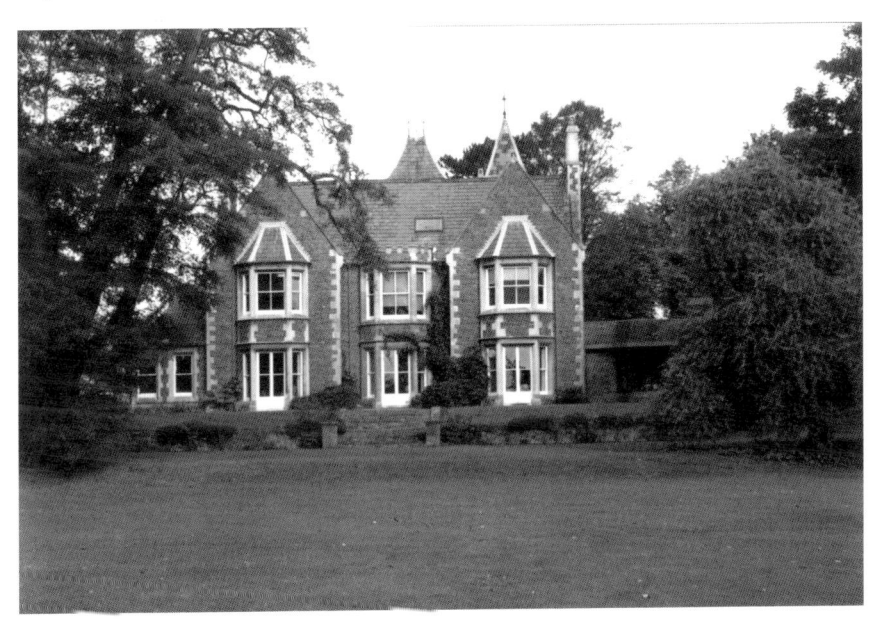

20. Priory Cottage 1997

This conflict between Miss Dallas' expectations for her students' training and the department's demands on the students meant that by 1966 the long-standing tradition of asking students to contribute to the social events for the residents in recognition of the lower than average fees was breaking down. Miss Dallas was said to have started to disapprove of the help given by her students at events such as barbecues and carnival parades, calling it 'a waste of time', even though the help was given in the students' own time. Sadly it seems that at about this time the student involvement in the pantomime ceases. Miss Dallas wrote a formal letter to the Hospital Administrative Officer, Mr. Heritage, to absolve her students from the duties of helping to decorate the wards at Christmas time. *'You will understand that the students in School have a complete lecture and practical programme which it is difficult to get through even without any interruptions to the number of hours they work.'*

On the other hand the staff in the hospital occupational therapy department who helped train the students, wrote a formal letter of complaint concerning the lack of organised support they were given by the School in the department's programme. Problems listed included the inadequate numbers of students on the wards and the fact that lectures sometimes were organised at the last minute and took priority over attendance on the wards. *'This has made programme planning difficult and has disrupted working rapport between patients, in addition to creating impossible situations between various members of the hospital team.'* Miss Dallas responded by suggesting to the Administrative Officer that the students' clinical practice be rearranged. *'Lectures, classes and holidays during the first five terms of training make it impossible for consistent attendance, and contact with patients is interrupted. It is felt that students should go on the wards during their final four terms, when regular lectures will have all been completed.'*

In 1966 circumstances seemed to be combining to hinder Miss Dallas' efforts to develop a harmonious prosperous School. She not only had to deal with the issue of her students' 'clinical practice' at the hospital, she had to deal with the problem of their accommodation. Even if formal clinical practice could be arranged at St. Andrew's in the final four terms, there were no arrangements in place to accommodate the students. There being no room in the second years' hostel, Miss Dallas had tried unsuccessfully to obtain rooms for them at the YWCA during the period when the School closed over the Summer. She had reluctantly agreed to allow the top floor bedrooms at Priory Cottage to be used even though there was no senior person living in who would be responsible for locking up etc. During term-time Miss Opsahl undertook this duty. Coupled with this, there had been no domestic staff at the School all through the summer term of 1966 owing to staff shortages. The summer holidays proved even more difficult to cover. Miss Dallas was away for a few weeks at the end of August, so for a while there was no one on hand to keep an eye on the students housed in the eerie top floor of Priory Cottage. One parent even felt obliged to write a letter of complaint to Mr. Heritage: *'The four girls have been quartered in a large lonely building ... The place was filthy dirty and they had to clean the bedrooms before they could be slept in. The bedroom doors could not be locked. This in the grounds of a mental hospital is hardly the way to ensure security.'*

The circumstances culminated in a potentially dangerous incident when the girls left the back door unlocked and found a male patient half naked in one of their bedrooms. The police were informed and one of the parents threatened to inform the press. Swift action to re-house the girls in other hospital accommodation helped to calm the situation, but not without the harassed Mr. Heritage declaring, *'Unless we can run the School properly, (and what staff Miss Dallas has to do this I do not know), it might be wise to close the School altogether and let it run down over a period of three years.'*

Miss Dallas's love of cats was almost the last straw in that fraught summer of '66. There were a number of cats roaming wild around Priory Cottage and students claimed that they had to feed them, often not being paid for the cost of the food. The staff saw it as yet another cause for complaint about the organisation of the School: *'We are constantly being approached by students resident at Priory Cottage and other hospital staff about the cats running wild, thus causing staff embarrassment in addition to embarrassment to visitors. The smell is very evident in Priory and in the surrounding grounds. Students are forced to feed the cats, often not recovering the cost of the food.'*

The School's idyllic surroundings of a beautiful Victorian villa and garden, set in the grounds of one of the foremost private psychiatric hospitals in the country began to look rather hollow. There were problems and difficulties which had to be addressed. The inspection that took place in March of 1966 exposed several other shortcomings, not just the ones relating to the organisation of clinical practice and domestic arrangements. The 1960s may have been a watershed decade for the occupational therapy profession, as suggested at the beginning of this chapter; 1966 was perhaps a watershed for St. Andrew's School.

Chapter 5

The Watershed

Elin Dallas 1957 –1972 (cont.)

1966 improvements to the School suggested, including greater emphasis on physical side of the therapy – Less emphasis on high standard of craftwork – Students learn about St. Andrew's new treatment for people with addictions – 1970 students appeal for more democracy at the School.

On March 15th1966 the School was visited by a team of five officials representing the A.O.T. and the State Registration Board. They acknowledged the pleasant atmosphere of the School and the teaching facilities at Priory Cottage, along with the well equipped occupational therapy department at Gloucester House. They also noted that the staff-student relationship appeared to be excellent. However, they made seven recommendations in the light of the pressures on the current staff and the inadequacies of the teaching on occupational therapy for physical disabilities:
1. The School should be separated from the hospital.
2. The Principal should be released from her duties as Head Occupational Therapist to the hospital.
3. A School Committee should be set up consisting of the Principal and representatives from a university, medical profession and the Committee of Management of St. Andrew's.
4. Teaching staff should be increased by two permanent members, one of whom should be Deputy Principal. In the event of the illness of the Principal no full-time staff would appear to be available under present arrangements.
5. A part-time secretary should be appointed to help with correspondence, filing timetables etc.
6. The Principal's salary did not appear to be on the recognised Whitley scale. This should be augmented as other staff's salaries were on either the Whitley or the Burnham scales.

7. Better facilities and equipment for teaching occupational therapy for physical disabilities should be provided as a matter of urgency.

The Medical Superintendent, Dr. O'Connell, retired shortly after the inspectors made their recommendations and his successor, Dr. Harper, was able to assure the Inspection board that the changes were being implemented. The staffing issues were being addressed and additional physical equipment was to be obtained. It was also hoped that local departments could be found, such as Kettering General Hospital, in which the students could obtain further instruction on the physical application of occupational therapy. The separation of the School from the hospital took place, but Dr. Harper's annual report does not suggest that much would change as regards the students' involvement with the patients. *'Close ties between the School and Hospital remain despite the administrative change. The School can take advantage of the teaching tradition of the hospital and its recreational facilities. The hospital benefits from the enthusiastic help of the students in the various social activities.'*

To accommodate the new equipment for physically disabled people (ADL) a room was taken over in the old nursing school at Wantage House and the apparatus was eagerly demonstrated to visitors on the following Open Day. The visitors were said to be very impressed. Items such as chair raisers and teapot tilters were new and exciting to the uninitiated. Four years later, in 1970, the ground floor of Priory Cottage had been opened up to provide a large kitchen space to aid in instructing the students on occupational therapy applied to physical disability. As a further improvement, links with supervisors at the various placements for clinical practice were more formalised so that regular meetings were organised, the supervisors visiting the School to learn more about what was required of them.

As far as domestic arrangements were concerned, the Hospital Board took a calm attitude to the flurry of parental complaints over Priory Cottage during the Summer of 1966. They merely commented that students should not have been living there unsupervised in the first place. (By 1969 the top floor was no longer used as a student residence. By then the absence of a fire escape meant that it was seen as a fire hazard.) Also, in 1967 for some reason that is not quite clear the School decided not to admit male students unless there were very exceptional circumstances, and reference to male students was deleted from the advertisements.

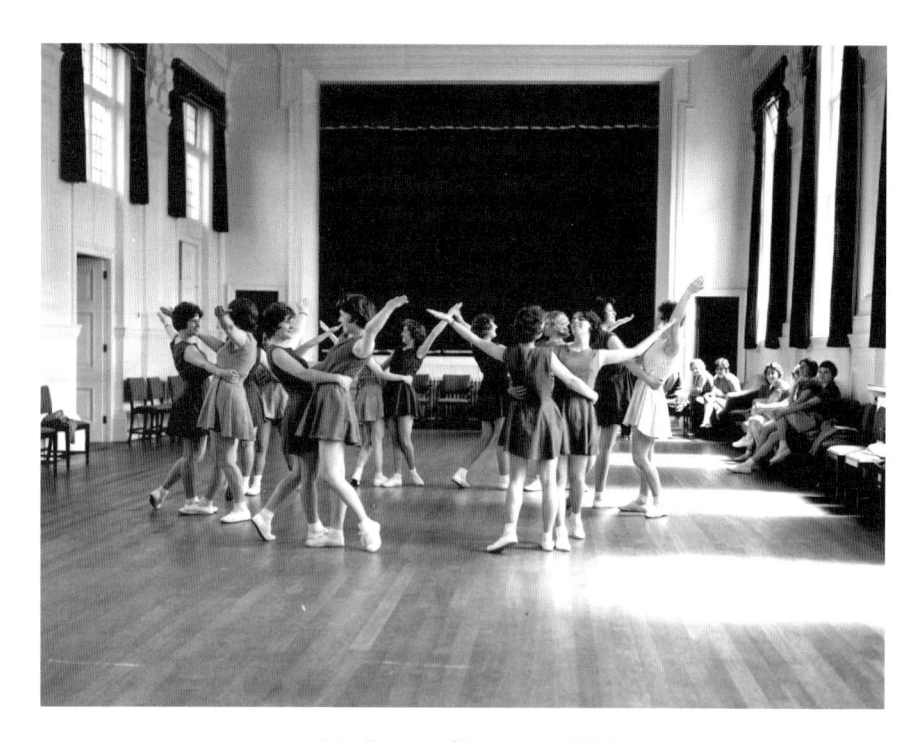

21. Dance Class ca. 1960

Most importantly staffing began to improve as the School was reorganised and separated from the hospital. A part-time secretary was not appointed until 1969, but Maria Van Garderen approached the School late in 1966 with a view to taking up the vacant post of Deputy Principal and began work in January the following year. She was Dutch and had been acting Vice Principal of the Liverpool College of Occupational Therapy. Remarkably different from Miss Dallas both in character and clinical experience, her story belongs in the next chapter for she took over from Miss Dallas in 1972. It must be said here, however, that she helped to bring the teaching up-to-date. Miss Dallas had been out of the profession for some time – as Head Occupational Therapist she had had little practical involvement with patients, and Maria Van Garderen was very keen on the latest theories and practice in the profession.

The new School Management Committee was set up quite quickly, including the Medical Superintendent, Dr. Harper, the Administrative Officer, Mr. Heritage, two hospital governors, Miss Dallas and Professor A. Allaway, who was Head of the Department of Adult Education at Leicester University. They took action to improve the finances of the School, observing in 1968 that the current profit of £260 was quite insufficient to enable any improvements to equipment and buildings. As a consequence fees went up by no less than one third. The large increase was partly justified as bringing the School in line with comparable schools. It is a sad indication of the effects of inflation at this time that within three years the fees were again significantly increased, by 25%. As well as increasing the fees the intake went up from 28 (in 1967) to 36 in 1968. Miss Dallas always took a few more students than she could easily accommodate because she had found that a few usually dropped out after the probationary term.

The selection of applicants to the School had in fact been considerably tightened up in 1967 because of the new exam policy brought in by the A.O.T. Only one re-take was to be allowed in Group I subjects (which were taken after the first year), a second one being only allowed in exceptional circumstances at the request of the Principal. The School introduced more frequent tests in the first six months in order to help discern those students who needed extra help and those who should be dissuaded from continuing. Miss Dallas was saddened to have to report this change in policy: *'In the School we have always persevered with students who found exams difficult but who were considered good in all other aspects. This may no longer be possible.'*

The new exam policy also included more freedom in interpreting the technical and recreational subjects on the syllabus, so that Housecraft, for instance, could mean cookery, curtain-making, or home repairs. By 1970 the syllabus had changed even more: the technical / recreational subjects became far less concerned with pure technique and were biased towards their use in group treatment. The emphasis was at last put on the application of the techniques rather than technical excellence. New subjects also were introduced such as splint-making and assessment of patients for ADL. This new bias in the syllabus reflects the trend which was referred to at the beginning of chapter 4 – the need for occupational therapists to be able to increase the independence of physically disabled people so that they could be discharged into the community. As the '60s drew to a close, St. Andrew's School found it was devoting more and more time to the physical aspects of occupational therapy rather than concentrating on the psychiatric side. In 1968 the students took part in a national project organised by the Central Council for Rehabilitation to survey the accessibility of public places for disabled people. Some of the students remember the novelty of the experience of going into town to carry out the survey: *'We went in a group with about two or three wheelchairs. It was really hard-going on the pavements and seeing how we'd get on and off them. We'd end up tipping somebody out. It was very difficult. It was quite dangerous and hard work if you were propelling yourself, and for the pusher particularly, with our capes getting tangled up in the wheels.'* In addition, the staff went on refresher courses on 'The problem of the disabled housewife in her kitchen' and 'Management of the severely disabled'. By 1971 the students were visiting various factories to analyse the work required and assess the working conditions with a view to reporting on the suitability of the factory for disabled people returning to employment.

The new syllabus now encouraged research projects to be undertaken. By 1969 there was already discussion about changing the diploma into a degree qualification for which independent research would be required, but the A.O.T. still favoured a more practical, less academic syllabus. The first PhD awarded to an occupational therapist was to Constance Owens at Liverpool in 1963, on the value of imagery in studying anatomy. On a national level research was being conducted on evaluating the design of rehabilitation equipment, and the first intervention trials on occupational therapy in the field of mental health were published in 1960. To practise their research skills students at St. Andrew's were choosing a variety of topics, such as the management of children with spina bifida and problems of communication in hemiplegia. The subjects are really essay topics rather than research, but it was early days. The standard of work was recognised as not what should be expected, but the intricacies of primary research were not yet being taught.

So by the end of the '60s the School had weathered the difficulties it had encountered in 1966 and once again looked forward to a promising future. Quite dramatic changes had been made in the School's relationship to the Hospital, for example, and it had begun to embrace the external changes taking place in the wider world of occupational therapy.

In 1970 the School was inspected for a second time in the four yearly cycle and this time it fared much better. In the recommendations it was noted that a second full-time member of staff had still not been appointed and that unless this was done, the intake should be reduced to a maximum of 20 students per year. Shortcomings in the teaching of anatomy and physiology were noted which could be improved with better coordination of teaching between the lecturer and tutor in these subjects. As far as the physical layout was concerned, it was suggested that the secretary have an office separate from the Principal's and that a staff room be made available. The clinical supervisors' meeting was not taking place as frequently as was to be expected; a recommendation was made for this to be an annual event. Links with the placements should also be

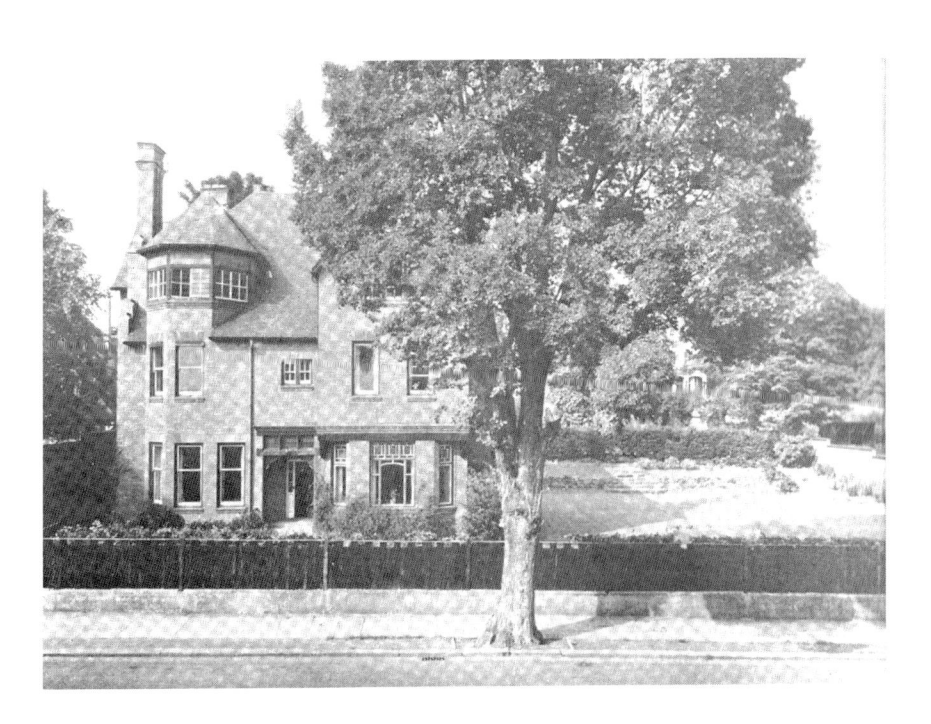

22. Lowood Student Hostel 1960s

improved, but it was recognised that visits by the School staff could only take place when additional staff had been appointed. One other major recommendation and one that reflects the new development taking place in the profession in general, was: *'There should be a reduction in time spent on weaving, drama, cord knotting, corn dollies, and an increase in time spent in Industrial Techniques, ADL, splints and commerce.'* The relationship between the staff and students was recognised as being very close, but the staff's attitude was viewed as being rather over-protective. The tutorial system of teaching was *'fairly rigid with an emphasis on note-taking and perfect folio reproduction ... There was not a great deal of evidence of active practical participation by the students.'*

In general, however, the outcome of the inspection was favourable; *'The general impression gained is of a very well run School with everything well organised, and with a character of its own ... The girls appeared confident, without being over confident, were pleasant as individuals and groups, enjoyed the experience of working with patients, and were well prepared for this part of their training. All students spoke with enthusiasm about their work and were clearly motivated to work hard.'*

The School may have changed during the 1960s both administratively and academically, but what kind of experience did the students have? How different was their time not just in the wider world out on clinical placements but in the social whirl of hostel life? Some of them recall the excitement and sense of freedom that came with the latest fashions of the Swinging Sixties – mini skirts, hot pants and PVC boots, and with the independence afforded by squeezing into a friend's mini on the way to the next disco, usually held in a village hall. The Conservative Club, situated close by on the corner of Cliftonville Road, proved an unlikely but lively source of company, as the YCs (Young Conservatives) met there and provided a ready made social life for the students living nearby.

In the hostels the warden, Miss Slater, felt as beleaguered as ever as she tried to curb the late night parties and candle burning. In February 1967 she wrote to Mr. Heritage to explain her frustration both at being unable to take adequate time off and at the way in which no disciplinary action was taken against students who broke the rules. Miss Dallas' 'severe reprimands' had no real effect. Also there was an acute domestic staff problem, two vacancies existing but with no applicants forthcoming. *'Nowadays I can no longer get staff to work on Saturday mornings – they all want a five day week. Therefore my Saturday mornings are spent doing every kind of domestic chore, including clearing out the hot water boiler and carrying coke from the cellar'* – a task the students and domestic workers would not do. Eventually two third year students were asked to live in at Kingswood and take on the duties of warden, thereby providing some assistance to the distraught Miss Slater. However, she still found her position hard. *'She hated any noise and prevented bedroom doors from closing completely (thereby stopping them from banging) by attaching an old stuffed stocking between the door handles of each door. If things got really bad, she wandered about complaining with a hot water bottle on her head to stop her head from aching.'*

The Eligibles Book continued, attendance at the annual ball still being compulsory and woe betide any girl who became engaged. *'They had all these silly rules, like you weren't allowed to be engaged. So if anyone did get engaged, they wore the ring round their neck on a chain.* Miss Dallas did not approve: "Training you and then you go and get married?" ' *'It was all hell let loose if someone got married. One girl got married one holiday and they stopped her training. She was out.'* This disapproval was in sharp contrast with the government's attitude to the 'cataclysmic' shortage of occupational therapists. In the 1960s they started to appeal to those who were married to return to work, and suggested ways in which this could be made possible – job sharing, flexible hours, free crèches and clinical refresher courses. As it was, of the practising membership of the A.O.T. only 47% of full-time staff were married and 58% of part-time. Of the non-practising members, 82% were married.

At the other end of the scale in this middle class world, several young Nigerian men entered the School during the 60s. Some of them came from very wealthy backgrounds, having been to the best school in Lagos and learnt English from English speaking tutors. Their experience of life in Northampton sometimes proved to be very hard. Linguistically they struggled with the grammar and the local accent. *'Being a black person among thirty odd white girls, it was difficult to fit in. Very difficult. The students and colleagues were wary. Some of them came from areas where they'd never seen a black person ... Finding digs was hard. Accommodation would be there. You'd go to see it and they'd look at you like this ... It wasn't just the School. The patients and staff of St. Andrew's were hostile – really hostile. There were also a lot of Caribbean nurses there, but it was terrible. You could go through hell.'*

Towards the end of the '60s, in common with the rest of the student population a certain militancy among St. Andrew's students became evident. In November 1970 they organised a working committee to plan an official student organisation 'to promote and maintain their views on problems in occupational therapy training as a whole'. They wanted there to be regular monthly meetings with the staff. Both Miss Dallas and Mr. Heritage were very against the idea, the latter declaring, *'Rather than put up with a militant student organisation I should prefer to see the School closed down, but perhaps I am exaggerating and meeting trouble half way. Our primary purpose is to run a hospital. The School is merely a welcome addition.'* Miss Dallas made some efforts to respond positively by asking other Heads of Schools for their experiences of this issue. However, it was finally pointed out to the students that as they were already members of the National Occupational Therapy Students Association and Students Union, no other organisation was deemed necessary.

In the wider world of clinical practice several students have said how glad they were to be able to see physical occupational therapy in practice, having merely encountered it at St. Andrew's in a small room containing a jumble of rehabilitation equipment. The students were also seeing the changing face of occupational therapy for themselves, once outside the somewhat rarified world of St. Andrew's. In the earlier years of the 1960s placements were provided at Napsbury, St. Crispin's, Edgware

General, the Medway Group, Farnham Park Rehabilitation Centre, and Passmore Edwards at Clacton. By 1965 there was a new placement at the Stoke Mandeville Polio Research Centre where severely disabled people were trained to use electronic ADL in order to achieve more independence. Then in 1969 students were given the opportunity to experience two very specific fields – the London Hospital Cerebral Palsy Unit and the Domiciliary Service of the London Borough of Hounslow Welfare Department. In the latter they were able to learn about how the new area of 'care in the community' worked. Some of the cases were of course physically disabled people. These were the days when the term 'handicapped' was still in use and there was a serious mood to improve the quality of lives and the independence of this group of people. It is interesting and amusing therefore to hear some of the reminiscences of one particular student of this period whose Irish sense of humour gave her a totally different attitude. *'People in Britain took it more seriously. I can remember talking to a group of young disabled people and I was in serious trouble because I told the story of this guy who was an amputee in Dublin. He was known for his denim jackets that always had something written on the back. The day I saw him, he'd written on the back "Legless but still sober". They didn't think it funny at all. They thought it was making a mockery. Another time I was working with someone in a wheelchair. He came in one day from the car park and it had been raining, and all down the corridor were dirty tyre marks. I said, "Oh Tim, you never wipe your feet, do you." Everybody was shocked, but Tim laughed. He knew what I was getting at.'*

Clinical placements in the area of rehabilitation brought students into contact with the new field of hand rehabilitation which was quite a recent specialised area of occupational therapy and one which students encountered at Medway and Farnham Park. The latter was particularly interesting for its industrial therapy. The rehabilitation centre was one of the first in the country and had been founded in 1947 by Mary Jones, who had done a lot of work adapting tools and equipment for patients at Rowley Bristow Hospital, Pyrford in the 1940s. Jones introduced the personal profit motive to prevent her patients feeling bored or exploited. Many of them were there because of industrial accidents or brain injury. One St. Andrew's student recalls how factories would set up a manufacturing outlet in the occupational therapy unit. The staff would base their treatment on that: *'You set up equipment to help with mobility of the ankle, for example – you had to work the equipment with your foot. We could also set up equipment with pulleys or slings to work the arm. We used to call it 'slings and springs' because you had so many springs against so many weights.'*

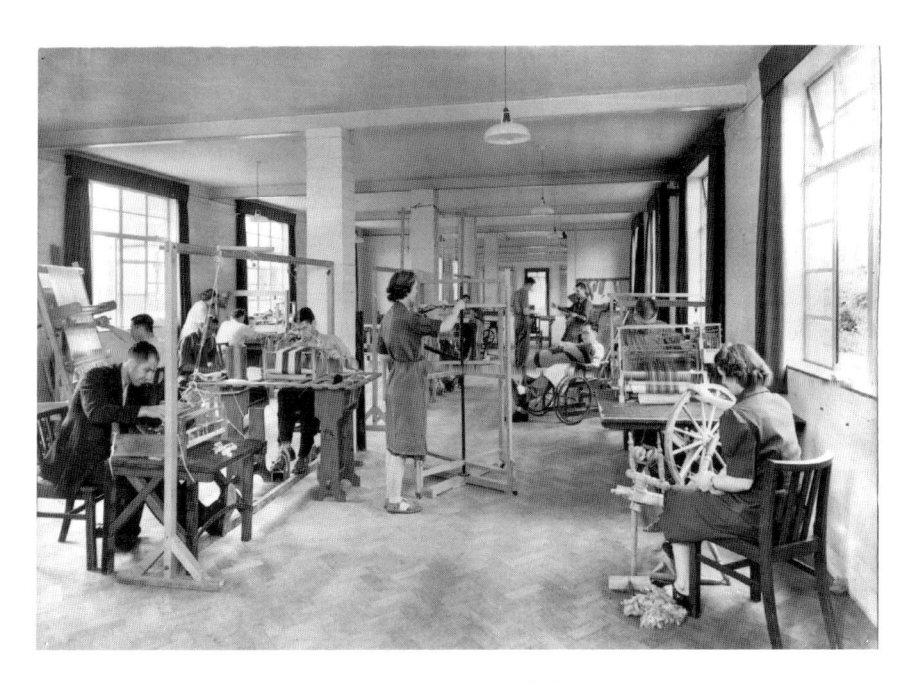

23. Manfield Orthopaedic Hospital OT Department 1950s

'People's jobs were totally different so you orientated yourself to what they had been doing before their injury ... You might have a bricklayer who'd broken his ankle. In the last stage of his treatment you'd have to take him out in his boots over muddy ground and do an activity that was using all the movements of his foot ... In the heavy workshops people might be doing woodwork at different height benches for their backs, or on lathes with their legs strung up if they'd had a knee injury ... People who'd had strokes or leg injuries and needed to improve their health generally would be on electric bicycles. At the same time they would be powering a treadle cutting something out of a piece of wood to make a model or a jigsaw. You could grade the height of the seat if you wanted them to do a certain movement involving the knee.'

Students at Medway worked with orthopaedic day cases and found that their knowledge of anatomy was thoroughly tested in the real world: 'You'd get somebody come in who'd had a fracture in the wrist and you'd have to know exactly what the problem was with their whole hand - what would have caused it. The Head Occupational Therapist, Miss Bell, would shout your name down the corridor and say, "Tell me all the muscles of extension in the fingers". You'd have to have a very thorough knowledge of anatomy.' In this context it is interesting to note the difference this same student has noticed in the present day training.

'Learning now at Occupational Therapy School is much more problem-based. So students will be given a problem and have to do the research around it. Whereas we were told what are the muscles of extension in the hand, nowadays you have to work out how you would approach the problem. We did it the other way round. I'm quite worried sometimes when I meet a student and talk to them about something quite fundamental and they haven't met it. Because the training is problem-based, if they encounter an unfamiliar diagnosis they just go into their problem-based mode and research it and so forth. We would have it all within us. Our anatomy, psychology and physiology was very strong. It gave me confidence when going into a clinic with a doctor. I would know what he was talking about.'

Manfield Orthopaedic Hospital was the local unit where for a time students could experience some very good physical rehabilitation. Another interesting change took place over the years (although Manfield itself is now no longer a hospital) - the occupational therapists used to spend a great deal of time adapting equipment to treat injuries, whereas nowadays *'a lot of things don't need treatment any more. The surgery is so minute that patients do not stay long. Physiotherapists will do any rehabilitation that's required. I think the growth in occupational therapy has been in medicine rather than in orthopaedics, where the recognition has come in the way occupational therapists treat strokes and the contribution they can make to arthritis – that's where the ADL come in. At Manfield we were involved in a treatment which was interesting and fun, but they don't do it now.'*

Sometimes poor placements had a certain value in the way they demonstrated what kind of occupational therapy to avoid. *'One place I went to, they were knitting dishcloths, and then the assistant was undoing them. That was just very, very bad practice. I was really disgusted by it. Luckily I moved out of that unit and went to work in the adolescent department which opened my eyes to another completely different type of occupational therapy – hanging around with teenagers and working out what their problems were.'*

The three other local placements apart from Manfield were of course St. Andrew's and for a time in the early days Creaton Tuberculosis Sanatorium and St. Crispin's. It had in fact been Mrs. Hombersley who started occupational therapy at Creaton, thereby giving her students a useful insight into purely diversional therapy. *'They were so bored. TB spines were on their backs all the time, sometimes for over twelve months. They didn't have antibiotics then (1945). The doctor must have*

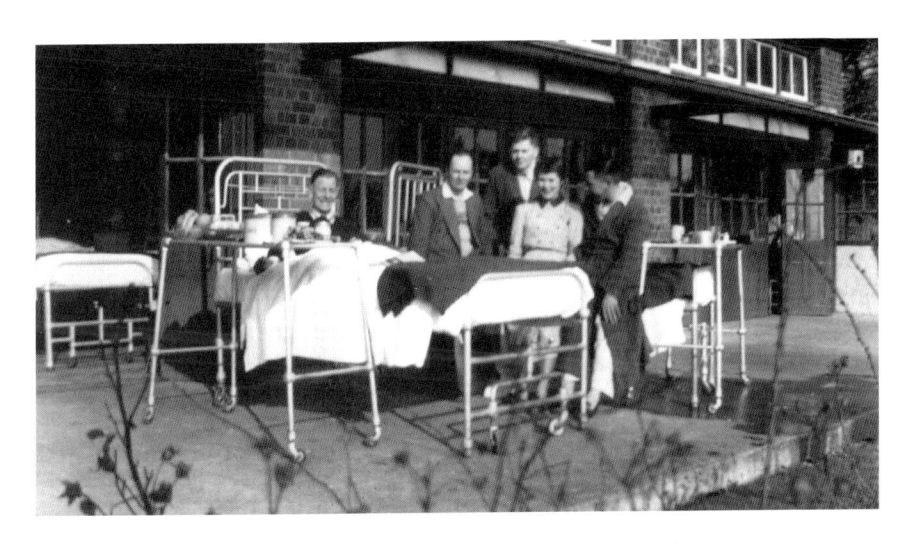

24. Creaton TB Sanatorium, in the garden

had a contact with the Air Force because we had old airmen's jackets with sheepskin linings. We could make slippers out of those. We had parachute silks. We even had old aeroplane wings that we could cut down to use the wood. We did an awful lot of recycling. We made lovely toys out the Air Force jackets. We used to go back in the evenings to do play readings with them. I encouraged them to write plays and we tried reading them. Sometimes they were good, sometimes they were terrible. If it was a fine day, no matter what the weather, we pushed the patients out of doors because they needed fresh air. It was a very interesting life in those days. It really was.'

On occasion quite complicated operations were performed at Creaton and afterwards patients had to do weaving with a long loom. This was a craft directly related to improving their lung capacity; the activity required a lot of stretching. Apart from TB there were polio cases. '*I was horrified when I saw my first polio patient in an iron lung. They couldn't do anything. It was up to us to set up a frame and page turner for them so they could look at a book. We had to be quite ingenious really.*'

Clinical work at St. Crispin's in the 1950s was quite a shock to students used to the up-to-date wealthy environment of St. Andrew's. '*The occupational therapy workshop was always quite lively, but going into the hospital with its dark brown walls up to head height and the patients who were drugged or very poorly was quite frightening. It smacked of Victorian times.*' ... '*St. Andrew's was always clean but St. Crispin's had certain smells. You never forgot the smells. Largactyl had a very sweet cloying smell – it was used for schizophrenia. The other smell was tobacco – gold cut to roll your own. It was particularly pungent. And urine. You'd go into a ward and the smells would hit you immediately.'*

Clinical practice at St. Andrew's itself was convenient for the students and of course gave a useful insight into the treatment of mental illness. One student from the late '50s appreciated the absence of medication among the patients. *'We were fortunate in a way that tranquillisers were only just coming in in the '50s and St. Andrew's was very reluctant to put them into use until they had been tried and tested. So we saw a lot of patients who had very florid symptoms which you don't see today – patients with very vivid visual hallucinations where they could obviously actually see whatever it was that was annoying them ... I remember at St. Andrew's you could smell the very crude drugs they used before tranquillisers came in. Unlike tranquillisers they'd make patients a bit like zombies and we'd see people in a catatonic state where they were just like a shop mannequin, frozen in one position and unable to move.'* Padded cells were still in use, even strait jackets, and despite the tranquillisers in use by the 1960s the students could still feel uneasy. *'On our first hospital practice we went on to a ward for the chronically ill and we all huddled into a corner feeling scared to death. One girl was very brave and went up to speak to a patient who said she was the queen of the butterflies. The patient sitting next to her just whammed this poor girl on the back. That made us even more scared of course.'*

Students had the impression, however, that St. Andrew's was unusual in that it was much more free and open than most psychiatric hospitals. *'They showed some Americans around the hospital on one occasion, and in one of the upstairs wards one of the American nurses said, "Gee, no bars on the windows. We have to have bars or they'd jump out." The member of staff showing them round said, "Do you know, we find if we leave the door open they prefer to walk down the stairs." That to me typified St. Andrew's attitude. The locked wards were very few and far between. There was a freedom at St. Andrew's. I think it worked both ways. People from Northampton were always very accepting. If patients were safe to go into town, then they went. The openness was there. I can remember one morning some of the patients were saying they had gone for a walk and seen lots of courting couples in the grounds. I really felt this shouldn't be allowed, but the doctor said that the big problem with access was that open gates open both ways. We couldn't expect to be able to go out into town and expect the townspeople not to come back in.'*

As the Mental Health Act came into force, there were several cases at St. Andrew's which came up for appeal with a view to allowing some of the long-stay residents to be cared for in the community. '*You wonder how many of the patients at St. Andrew's should have been there. One lady in particular I remember. She'd been there 22 years and she told me that as a teenager she'd fallen in love with the wrong man. She was from an aristocratic family who'd disapproved of him. He was sent off and she went into a manic depression – didn't eat or sleep - and so she ended up at St. Andrew's. I would say a lot of patients there were more eccentric than mad.*' This same student is amused to recall how the students could find themselves going along with the various eccentricities. '*I had a conversation with a lady – she was very concerned about what was going to happen to her body when she died. Her family wanted her to be buried with her father in Zurich, but she got seasick. I found myself – the sane one – saying, "I'm sure it won't matter if you fly". That's what St. Andrew's did to you!*'

It was during the '60s that the hospital began to treat alcoholics and drug addicts. One student remembers the aversion therapy that was used to try to wean people off alcohol and how it didn't always work. Of course addicts could be mentally very bright and show great ingenuity, presenting the students with different problems from those of the mentally ill. '*In the late '60s there was a very big group of young drug addicts. They took this fantastic interest in pottery, so I left them to it. One of them came into the office and said they'd finished the pottery and could they fire it. I said yes and went out to see. They'd produced hundreds of chillums, which were the pipes used to smoke hash. They were going to go down to Piccadilly and make a fortune selling these pipes. I didn't fire them, believe me! ... It was very sad to see what heroin does. One young man said he would rather die. We said to him "Do you realise you're not going to last long?" and he said, "I'd rather die at 21 on heroin than live a long life without it." That was terribly sad.*'

The clinical placement part of the curriculum was clearly an important experience for the students and one of which the students have both good and bad memories. The lack of organised supervision, noted in the School inspection of 1966, may have meant that they did not always learn as much as they might have, but the third years always came back to their final term with a wealth of experience on which they could draw in their future careers. Miss Dallas even noticed that they came back with more than just memories: '*When she was introducing one set of third years to the new Vice Principal, Miss Van Garderen, she asked that they be kind to her. "Third years are very frightening. You've all got your hospital walks now and you're frightening, so be kind to Miss Van Garderen."'*

Miss Dallas retired in 1973. She had brought to the School many distinctive qualities such as the use of dance and drama as an important part of occupational therapy, and the introduction of beauty therapy. Her students went out on a growing number and variety of clinical placements where they often learnt to realise one of the most distinguishing features of their School: - when they compared notes with their student colleagues they seemed fortunate in the amount of patient contact which they were able to enjoy at St. Andrew's. The School may not always have been as well organised, both domestically and academically, as it could have been, but results remained good and the School flourished in terms of the number of applications. The inspection of 1966 served to help put the School on a more viable footing, economically and academically.

As has been mentioned above, the emphasis on craft work was just beginning to be reduced as the 1960s drew to a close, but the profession was still undergoing difficulties as it struggled to promote its image to a rather ignorant and bemused public. One student remembers with typical exasperation '*We were always having to say what occupational therapy was and explain ourselves to the non-medical professions and to the patients. And basketry became a joke, but was a little difficult because basketry was one of our activities. Somebody would say, "Did you learn to make baskets?!" and you had to say, yes, you had. It was actually very good for people who'd had breast cancer – as just one example. I think its use just went overboard.*'

In face of the difficult circumstances of staff shortages and lack of available experience in physical rehabilitation, Miss Dallas continued to lead a School of which it seems most of her students have very fond memories. The last word should go to Miss Dallas herself. Like Mrs. Hombersley before her, by 1972 she knew her students were going out into a world where they would face obstacles and difficulties, if not lack of understanding. At her last graduation ceremony before retiring she gave some words of advice to her students which served to strengthen and inspire them in their still evolving profession - in a world where they might encounter disagreement from doctors, opposition even from patients and strange and bizarre behaviour. '*I want you all to remember that you are now occupational therapists. You will need three qualities – single-mindedness, humility and a sense of humour.*'

Chapter 6

A Step too far?

Maria Van Garderen 1972 – 1981

Growing political and industrial unrest – Rising inflation - A.O.T becomes a trade union – The new social model of disability - 1970 Chronically Sick and Disabled Person Act – Emphasis in occupational therapy on Aids for Daily Living – Introduction of multi-disciplinary teamwork into the profession - 'The decade of self-doubt'.
Growing rebelliousness among students – NHS students receive DHSS awards instead of LEA grants – National shortage of occupational therapy teaching staff reaches crisis point – A.O.T. introduces clearing house system - Small increase in number of mature students and growing variety of social backgrounds.
Schools given new freedom to design and assess their own diplomas – Education methods evolve, including social skills group work – Schools start to become part of Polytechnics and Colleges of Higher Education.

The arrival of Maria Van Garderen in 1972 (or VG as she became known) signalled a change in direction for the School. She was much more experienced in the physical side of occupational therapy than Miss Dallas. *'She was Dutch and was very solid ... I can't imagine Dilly holding a plane or a saw as VG would have done ... She was very precise and very practical. She wore thick stockings, long tweed skirts, twin sets, with her grey hair scraped back and no make-up – very traditional and old-fashioned.'* Some of her students remember being petrified of her. She had quite an authoritarian style, at least on the surface, but by 1974 they had begun to be vocal in their complaints about the 'lack of domocracy' in the School. This minor rebellion in itself is an interesting reflection of the way in which students had begun to change. It is of course linked to wider developments in society as a whole. However, the 1970s saw more than a change of attitude and expectations among students; the health

77

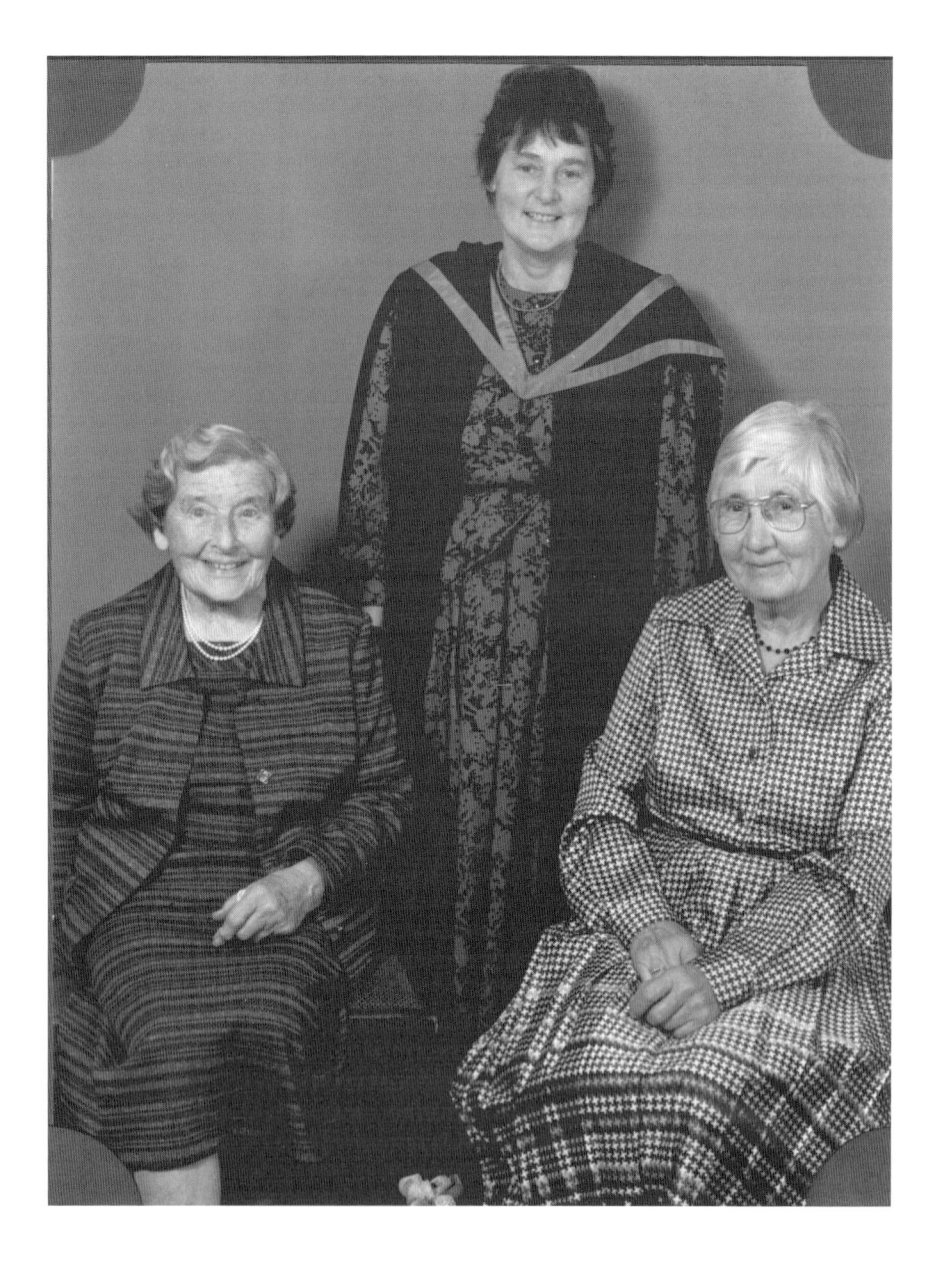

25. Three Directors of Training ca. 1990
Elin Dallas, Elizabeth Cracknell, Maria Van Garderen

service and occupational therapy profession were also evolving.

The change towards community rather than institutional care accelerated. More and more occupational therapists were being employed by local authorities to carry out functional assessments on physically disabled people and make provision for aids to help them live in their own home.

The structure behind the profession was also changing. In 1974 the A.O.T. joined with its Scottish counterpart, the S.A.O.T., to form the B.A.O.T. (British Association of Occupational Therapists) and eventually became a trade union, the C.O.T. (College of Occupational Therapy) being its wholly owned subsidiary to maintain the educational and professional aspects of the profession. The Casson Memorial Lecture was set up in 1971 to provide a stimulating platform for new ideas; the first European Congress on Occcupational Therapy was held in 1977, and awards of Fellowships were established by the B.A.O.T., partly to encourage research, but also to raise the profile of the profession. By the end of the decade new types of courses were being introduced – qualifications for occupational therapy helpers and post-registration courses, and the profession had been given a presence in government. This enhancing of the status of the profession can of course only have been for the good, but seems to have been particularly timely in an era when BBC Radio could include such comments as the following: '*An occupational therapist is one who stops people going crazy from boredom in hospital and also works in long-stay geriatric hospitals and with children.*' (Dr. Donald Gould)

The radio programme led to outrage among the profession – a reaction which recurred when discussion began in 1972 on the possibility of providing just one basic training course for physiotherapists, occupational therapists and remedial gymnasts, to be followed by a specialised programme within a new 'remedial profession'. The McMillan Committee set up a working party in 1973 to work out the ideal structure for this remedial service. The essence of the profession's reaction was expressed by Professor Cairns Aitken in his Casson Memorial Lecture of 1976. He feared that the value of occupational therapy was not being recognised and that physically disabled people were just being given cash benefits and not provided with the complementary professional services. He referred to occupational therapists' fears that their practical skills and the value of their skills in building relationships with people were insufficiently recognised. At one of the annual conferences of this period, Dr. J. Muir made a rousing speech in which he referred to what has become known as 'the social model', as opposed to 'the medical model' of disability – i.e. one in which disability is seen as caused by society rather than as a disease to be cured. *'Occupational therapists must be revolutionaries: physical disability has five main diseases – poverty, bad housing, being cold, (a lack of) independence in the home, and isolation. Occupational therapists must change society to prevent handicap being caused for people with disabilities, who are often unable to effect changes themselves.'* Already government legislation was being influenced by this new social model when in 1970 the Chronically Sick and Disabled Persons Act introduced the legal requirement that all public buildings should be accessible to disabled people.

The stirring words of Dr. Muir may not sound like the words of a profession in the throes of self-doubt, but that is precisely how the 1970s are perceived by Ann Wilcock in her history. As has already been seen at the end of the previous chapter on the 1960s, occupational therapists felt misunderstood not only by the general public but also by the medical fraternity. Wilcock suggests that the introduction of work on ADL may have been too rapid a change in direction for the profession. It seemed to entail a rejection of the old practices where illness was remediated by using craft work and recreational or vocational employment. The philosophical base for occupational therapy was being lost. The image of this relatively new profession has already been described here as fragile and uncertain in the 1960s. In the following decade there was evidence of a real sense of doubt about where occupational therapy was heading.

Closer to home, amid all these changes the St. Andrew's School was in a way cocooned by the modern development of the hospital's occupational therapy facilities. In 1971 the Medical Director declared that facilities for treatment could now be said to be 'adequate'. He was referring to the opening of the new Occupational Therapy Centre, the Industrial Therapy Unit and the Geriatric Occupational Centre. The School was indeed fortunate in having on its doorstep so many good examples of psychiatric occupational therapy. This sense of being cocooned is born out by the way in which the 1975 inspection report described the School as being 'educationally isolated'. At the beginning of the 1970s it seems the School was indeed only just beginning to get to grips with the need to expand its horizons both in the physical aspect of occupational therapy and in the search for a link with a local institute of higher education. In actual fact, up to 1975 Northampton only had a Teacher Training College and separate Technical and Arts Colleges. The former was at Moulton Park and the latter at St. George's Avenue. It was not until 1975 that Nene College was formed, uniting all three and providing a possible local link for the School.

Miss Van Garderen knew the changes which the profession was facing and she achieved a great deal in improvements to the School's facilities and curriculum and in the reduction of the drop-out and failure rates among her students. However, first of all the School's financial position had to be strengthened and the staffing issue addressed. In 1971 fees had been compared with other Schools and consequently increased significantly during the course of the decade – sometimes by as much as a quarter or a third each year. By 1977 the School Management Committee announced that the School was on a satisfactory footing financially and the fees for 1978 only increased by 10%. It was fortunate that since the School's separation from the hospital the latter was making no charge for the repairing lease of Priory Cottage. From the mid 70s the School no longer received a subsidy from the hospital.

The intake increased during VG's time so that from 32 in 1970 and 40 in 1978, there was a proposal to take 60 students in 1980. Not only did attention need to be paid to the adequacy of the fees, the students' grants had to be secured. This was achieved when in 1976 changes in government policy meant that all students in the NHS professions received DHSS awards rather than LEA grants.

The School was improving its facilities during the 1970s. The ADL room in Priory Cottage was too cramped, so the equipment was transferred to a more spacious flat within the hospital which became known as 'the flat for training towards independence'. A medical library opened in the hospital grounds and here the students had the benefit of a section on occupational therapy and a part-time librarian (apart from the reference library in Priory Cottage). The new medical library provided 16 individual study booths suitable for audio-visual self-teaching packages. The lecture hall was becoming over-crowded with the increase in students, and by 1979 discussions were being held on the possibility of the hospital extending Priory Cottage to provide a larger lecture hall and some seminar rooms.

The School did not just need to improve its physical resources; human resources were of course vital to its success. When Miss Van Garderen took over there was still a shortage of staff. Two important innovations were made to ease the problem – firstly, student teachers were employed and secondly, links were set up with Nene College.

In 1971 advertisements for two full-time staff had failed to attract any suitable applicants. The shortage of teaching staff in Occupational

Therapy Schools was said to have reached crisis point across the whole country. VG took decisive action to find a solution to the problem and in 1972 decided to train her own staff. She arranged a course of study at St. Andrew's for the Teacher's Diploma with help and advice from Leicester University and Nene College of Education, and obtained approval from the examining board. The first year exam was to be on Psychology and the second year, on the Principles and Practice of Teaching. Two students were thus taken on, providing teaching under Elin Dallas' supervision. The post of Deputy Director of Training was not so easily filled. The advertisement was placed overseas as well as in the UK but attracted no applications. It was therefore decided to increase by two the number of student teachers doing in-service training. Elin Dallas, although retired now, agreed to carry on as their tutor.

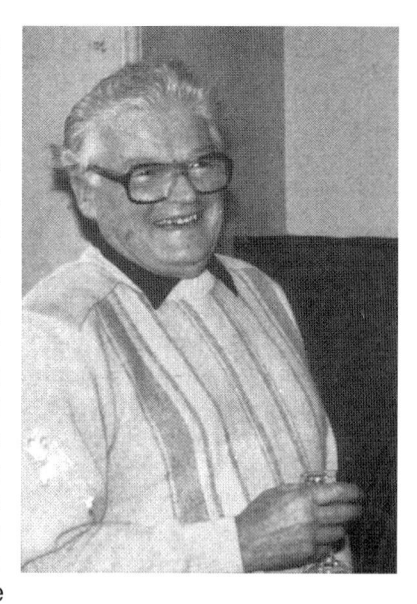

26. Neville Parsons Jones ('PJ')

However, the staffing and organisation of the School was not to go smoothly. 1974 saw a minor rebellion that disturbed the outwardly happy atmosphere. The competence of the young staff was not always satisfactory, leading to complaints from the students. Continuous assessment had been introduced, proving extremely unpopular. One well-liked member of staff decided to resign. 25% of 2nd year students left. A study carried out in 1978 noted that an average of 24% of students dropped out between 1967 and 1975. Whatever was going on nationally, the School suddenly seemed to have a rebellion on its hands when 56 students addressed a letter to Mr. Heritage on the School Management Committee listing ten grievances. One of the issues was that they were finding it difficult to accept Miss Van Garderen's strict manner in running the School. They cited her 'authoritarian ways' as the possible reason why staff and students were leaving. They even felt that 'the continuous assessment system is being used to intimidate people against voicing their opinions'. They complained about out-dated teaching methods, a lack of communication between the Principal, staff, students and the hospital, and that unsuitable clinical practices were being used. They also wished to have more opportunities for working in the hospital itself. As a result of this letter the School Management Committee agreed that more full-time staff would solve a lot of the problems, enabling the students to have tutorial groups (on which they were very keen) and enabling Miss Van Garderen to spend more time consulting with her staff and communicating with the School in general.

In 1978 Averil Stewart, the Educational Development Officer for the C.P.S.M. (Council for Professions Supplementary to Medicine) conducted a national survey of occupational therapy teaching resources in the UK. She spent a lot of time observing at all Schools and it is interesting how at St. Andrew's she sensed the difficulties which VG had been through, describing the episode as *'a recent period of restlessness and low morale'*. VG did seem to have a difficult year in 1974 to rival Miss Dallas' 1966. There was another inspection to prepare for in 1975, with all the concomitant paperwork, and she still did not have a deputy. After receiving the C.P.S.M. inspectors' report of 1975 the Committee at last appointed Hazel Starmer as the new Vice-Principal, and discussions were held about introducing a tutorial system despite the timetabling problems foreseen. Miss Van Garderen even started holding weekly meetings with her staff to improve communication and consultation. This was extended to include daily meetings over morning coffee in her office, although the system was noted by Averil Stewart to be less than successful – in fact, somewhat fraught. *'This does not seem to allow for informal and relaxed exchanges at all levels, and while the staff are supportive of each other, there are suggestions that within the staff group as a whole there is a lack of interest and understanding of the needs of each other – personal and workwise. The staff group would welcome a regular, perhaps monthly, less structured meeting for the exchange of ideas.'* In this regard it is worth noting that by 1980 weekly staff meetings were being held to discuss issues such as organisation, training, the syllabus, curriculum and assessment.

By the mid 70s at last a full complement of qualified staff was in place – two full-time and two part-time, enabling the School to take a maximum of 40 students per year. The increase in staff had made it possible to introduce an orientation course for the first years. New students, assigned to a particular tutor, divided into five groups and followed six weekly courses over a six week period, covering basic craft techniques and recreational activities, with introductions to academic and applied subjects. Time was allowed for the students to observe workers at their jobs and to consider the implications of different social environments. It was hoped the overall general introduction to occupational therapy would help the new students settle in and get to know their tutor.

If the immediate staffing issue was being addressed, what of the link with Nene College? In the summer of 1976 the Dean of the School of Sciences at Nene, Mr. D. George, approached the School with the offer to help teach the academic subjects of Anatomy, Physiology, Psychology and Sociology. The School's existing anatomy tutor, Miss Jennings, wanted to retire, so the offer was gratefully accepted. It was recognised of course that there would be additional benefits to the students in the wider facilities of Nene – a large library and students' union for example, and that the School would be able to save money on tuition. The students attended Nene one day a week and the Principal of the College, Dr. Ogilvie, was invited on to the School Management Committee. It took a while for the students to settle down at Nene. At first they found themselves in overcrowded portakabins with the Nene lecturers criticising their syllabus, and the timetable for Anatomy and Physiology proving too dense. As it turned out, results in these subjects did not improve, extra coaching needing to be provided back at the School. One year the thirteen re-sit students in Anatomy and Physiology were given a six week revision course in May and June instead of their first main clinical practice. The intensive coaching and threat of having to leave the course produced a 100% pass rate.

In 1978 the C.P.S.M. Study by Averil Stewart noted that the School's failure rate in academic exams was on or below the national average in all but Communication and Management. (Craft skills attained at the School were still higher than average.) The staff-student ratio of 17:1 was too high, but it was found that results were not related to the number of teaching hours; they probably reflected the teaching methods used. This issue was not properly addressed until several years later. On a practical level, matters improved at Nene, with classrooms being enlarged and the Psychology and Sociology lectures being moved to Priory Cottage, although in 1979 students were still complaining about the lack of transport to Nene (bicycles were no longer the norm as in the early days) – the bus service was proving less than adequate.

So as far as staffing was concerned, the link with Nene was providing some respite for the tutors at the School. Eight consultants from Northampton General Hospital were also on the part-time staff, providing lectures on Medicine, Surgery and Psychiatry, and by 1979 two more staff were taken on, one a student teacher and one a part-time clinician at St. Andrew's. Staff were also being given the opportunity to undertake further study, one tutor for example, beginning a three year degree for members of the remedial professions at the Polytechnic of Central London. Training was also started for clinical supervisors to improve the students' experience on clinical placements. In 1980 Miss Van Garderen organised a Basic two day Course at St. Andrew's which was attended by 30 occupational therapists. A five day Intermediate Clinical Supervisors' Course was provided one year later.

In general however, it is worth noting the comments made by Averil Stewart in her Study: *'It is difficult to establish standards and expectations through lack of contact with other education institutions ... Sitting in on lectures, visiting other Schools, attending management courses, participating in tutor group meetings and working for degrees, would all help towards increased effectiveness and morale.'*

While Miss Van Garderen was working hard to improve the staffing and teaching at the School, the alarming matter of the high drop-out rate also had to be tackled and she did this in a very methodical way by introducing psychological testing of applicants. Back in 1973 one student remembers being accepted on to the course even though she only had one 'F' at A-level. (Admittedly this was an exception – two A-levels were normally required.) In 1975 the AH4 Psychological Test was introduced, administered after two interviews, one with the Principal and one with the Vice-Principal. Candidates were also told that they had to visit an occupational therapy department before attending for interview. In its 1978 Study report the C.P.S.M. was very keen that Schools monitor the results of this AH4 test and interviewers' comments, comparing them with a student's later achievements. It was clear that nationwide the selection procedure needed to be made more effective. As more and more school leavers became interested in further study, it became not only more difficult to select the right candidates but also more important not to waste time and money training unsuitable students. At St. Andrew's applications for a place on the course had gone up so much that by 1978 five to six interviews were being held three times a month and Open Days held once a term. The new B.A.O.T. system of Clearing was introduced in 1977 and In the first year of operating it had produced so many applicants that the School had felt overwhelmed and returned over half without offer of an interview. The following year 138 applications were received via this route, of which 77 were selected for interview. Of these 42 were chosen.

The more thorough selection procedure did seem to have an effect, for in 1977 the drop-out rate in the first year reduced to 5% compared with an average between 1967 – 75 of 14.5%. However, in 1980 VG was dismayed to have to report a 15% drop-out again (7 out of 45), either because of exam failure, medical reasons or the wrong choice of career. She suggested that the answer might be to have better career education. Averil Stewart had made some interesting observations on the subject of 'wastage': She thought that although the problem was diminishing as the majority of students valued the opportunity to train for a profession, the number who showed a marked lack of interest probably reflected the new pressure applied to school leavers to go on to further study whether they wanted to or not. She also feared that the diploma course might not be sufficiently demanding and stimulating for the more intelligent students: *'Many are not given the opportunity to think for themselves and be flexible.'* In St. Andrew's she feared that *'individual members of staff experience conflict between wanting to give the students more freedom and opportunity for responsibility, at the same time maintaining control to ensure success in training'.*

One of the most important changes which Miss Van Garderen oversaw was in the area of the curriculum. The 1978 Study reported that the course was said to have *'changed tremendously since the Principal took over and that there is a constant search for improvement'.* Her introduction of one topic in particular in 1974 epitomises what she brought to the School in terms of her experience in occupational therapy for the physically disabled. The students were to receive twenty lectures in the course of the year on 'Gardening for the Disabled', for which appropriate tools were to be bought. Mr. White, who was in charge of national research in the subject, was invited to come and lecture. The course was very detailed, with a lecturer being invited in from Moulton College to teach horticulture and even agriculture. On a more general level a variety of visits were organised for the second years, one of which was to the new permanent exhibition of ADL at the Disabled Living Foundation. The courses and visits reflect VG's interest in expanding the students' experience of the physical side of occupational therapy. They did factory–type work locally at St. Andrew's, the Cliftonville Adult Training Centre and Nordis Sheltered Workshop. Visits were made to Avon Cosmetics and the Chronicle and Echo Printing Works, to Hinwick Hall School for Boys with Muscular Dystrophy, and to individuals' houses. One belonged to a person with cerebral palsy who used aids with patient-operated selector mechanisms; another, to a person using a wheelchair whose home benefited from various adaptations. The students were taught about the teamwork involved in rehabilitation, being given a talk by a panel consisting of a community occupational therapist, an architect for the Northampton Development Corporation and an officer from the Environmental Health department. This was a very useful and dramatically new approach to the concept of 'multi-disciplinary teamwork', bringing together people from such diverse backgrounds.

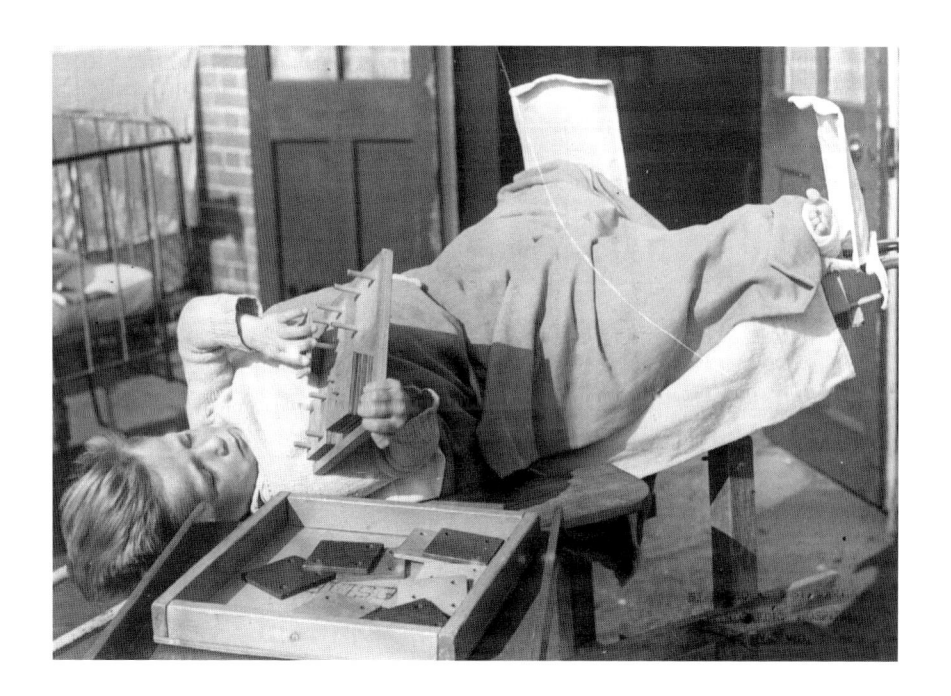

*27. St.Nicholas & St.Martin's Orthopaedic Hospital Pyrford,
Occupational therapy for a child*

Apart from improving the teaching on the physical side, Miss Van Garderen also oversaw a revision in the syllabus in 1974. Viva exams were phased out and the idea of continuous assessment introduced. Clinical supervisors' reports were now to form part of the final exam. More importantly the concept of the Internally Assessed and Externally Moderated (IAEM) curriculum was introduced, although at first it only affected Part I of the diploma. This enabled Miss Van Garderen to draw up her own Psychology and Sociology syllabus, which she completed with the help of her staff and external lecturers. The final Part I exam in the summer was to be coupled with an essay in the Spring term. Approval was obtained from the C.P.S.M. and B.A.O.T. An external moderator had to attend the School to check on the validity of the results.

Once the new syllabus was in place, Miss Van Garderen set to work to plan new Anatomy and Physiology courses, intending to concentrate on functions of the body rather than detailed knowledge of the structure. Students must have been very pleased to hear of the impending change, although some may have feared that they had wasted their time learning by rote for a career where such detailed knowledge would not be required. *'We could name every bone, nerve, muscle extension – we could repeat it over breakfast. It was very scientific.'* This particular student observed that in the early 70s the medical model of disability was still very much in evidence. The doctor was always in charge. The kind of work that the occupational therapists did, based on anatomy and physiology, would later be undertaken by physiotherapists.

Along with these new courses Miss Van Garderen introduced a series of special weekly lectures for the second years, examples of which included Mental Subnormality, Occupational Therapy with Elderly Patients, the Assessment Unit of the Princess Marina Hospital for the Mentally Subnormal and the Work of a Clinical Psychologist. The third years and staff were able to benefit from the introduction of post-exam courses such as the ones on Bobath Techniques and Creative Therapies.

As far as the practical curriculum was concerned, the School still devoted quite a large part of the timetable to crafts and their professional application. The 1978 Study provides useful insight into the staff's attitude. Evidently prior to the 1978/9 academic year fears had been expressed that there was an over-emphasis on craft subjects and some subjects needed to be ruthlessly pruned from the curriculum. The danger was recognised that students were being taught a little about too much: *'There is a danger that newly qualified occupational therapists, having tasted so many, feel secure with none; standards are unknown; they seek refuge in assessment forms and in fact use less treatment techniques.'* It was noted in the Study that the School had not yet done much to alter the timetable despite these concerns. On the other hand, this attitude towards craft work was not a total rejection of its value either by the staff or the profession in general. Ann Wilcock points out in her history that in the 1970s crafts were being reintroduced to some hospital departments because they were found to be useful for such things as retraining concentration after a brain injury, learning manipulation after nerve lesions, and preparation for the world of work. One student from the mid 70s does feel that there was a tendency nationally to reject craft work out of hand: *'The craft that we were brought up with, was suddenly seen as a bit of a taboo subject. It did go through that reputation of being just basket weaving ... so we had to become more scientific. A lot of these craft activities were thrown out, which is a shame in some ways because they were just thrown out without any reason as to why.'*

There is another interesting aspect of this movement away from craft activity. Perhaps it was only just beginning at the School in the 1970s, but it was to become an important part of occupational therapy,

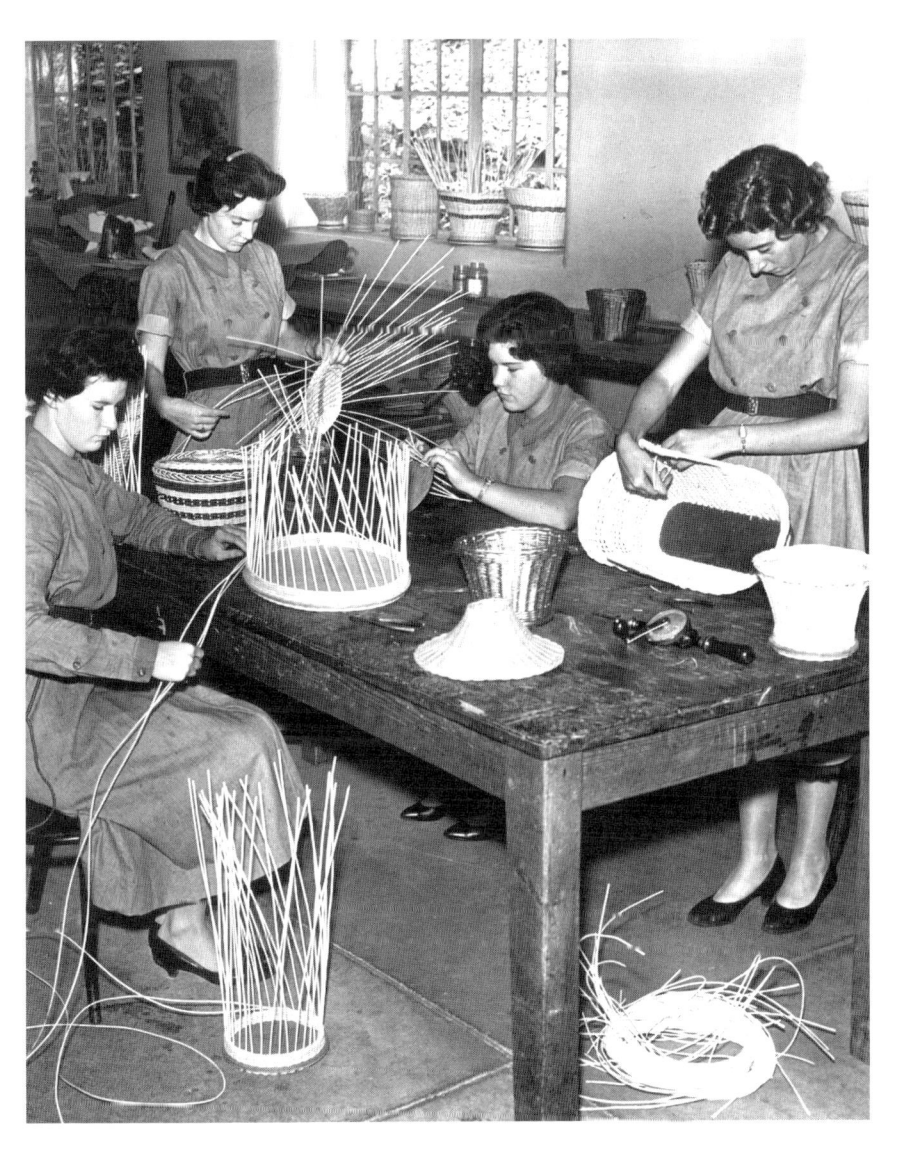

28. Basket making

especially in mental health. One of the students from this period suggests, *'We were the beginning of the generation who were trying to get rid of the basket weavers and the arty farty image ... A lot of the stuff in mental health that we were doing was group work – things like social skills groups, social interaction – talking-type groups as opposed to activity groups … There was that idea that occupational therapists occupied people … We were trying to shake that image off. I think even as students we felt it.'*

It is interesting to note that the balance towards the physical side which Miss Van Garderen had sought to redress, seemed to have swung too far the other way. Averil Stewart noted in the School *'an imbalance between Physical and Psychiatric, with more time being spent on Theory in Physical.'* Students were doing a lot of work on ADL. They were fortunate in being given the chance to help a local domiciliary occupational therapist make or adapt equipment for her clients. Small groups would go out into the community to meet users of the service and sometimes these users would come into the School. This programme of activity continued for quite a few years, but as the number of students increased, the logistics of transporting clients in and out became too complicated and unfortunately it came to an end.

Towards the end of Miss Van Garderen's time as Principal students were spending a lot of time just practising techniques - learning how to hoist up a client, help them into a wheelchair, teach them to walk up- and downstairs, even adapt a toilet. This was part of their course on Adaptive Equipment which encouraged them to think creatively in order to solve a problem. Interestingly one current tutor has pointed out that fear of litigation precludes current students from daring to modify a piece of equipment for a disabled person.

Physical recreation, although not mentioned in the 1978 Study, still featured in the curriculum up to the mid 70s and was now taught by Mrs. Kempston, a former ballet dancer. Apart from learning dancing, ballgames and other sport, the students were drilled in deportment. *'We had to learn to sit right; we had to learn how to curtsey; we had to learn when we sat on the floor where our legs were … You'd think more people would have rebelled. I mean students now would just laugh their heads off. They would just fall about laughing, but we all did it. It was early days and we were all just 18 or 19, so we just took it all in. Prim and proper and ladylike – even if you weren't.'*

The students still benefited from the proximity of the hospital and the daily contact with the patients, whether just going for meals in the canteen or working with them in one of the social activities such as the pantomime or an evening of board games. When Miss Van Garderen took over as Principal she reported that with the increase in School staff and the improved facilities for training, it was now possible to integrate more with the occupational therapy department at the hospital. No less than eleven students per year did their clinical practice at St. Andrew's, and in 1976 places were even being offered to students from Dorset House, enabling a healthy exchange of ideas. It is as well to remember, however, that the use of St. Andrew's for placements was not enough integration as far as many of the students were concerned. The minor rebellion in 1974 culminating in a letter to the School Management Committee revealed that they wanted more work with the patients. *'The sad fact is that even though the School is situated in the grounds of one of the leading psychiatric hospitals of this country, we have little opportunity of benefiting from this.'* In the 1978 Study the situation did not seem to have changed greatly, but it was felt that *'many opportunities are created for contact prior to clinical practice.'* Perhaps the timetable just could not sustain the amount of clinical work which the first year students desired, although parties, quizzes, tennis matches, whist drives and plays all feature in the reporting of events at the School.

It seems that most of the students, whether on a placement or just in daily contact, learnt to enjoy the various eccentricities which they encountered, even if they did occur at very inopportune times: *'When I took my final papers, we were in the great hall and a well-known character comes in and starts playing on the grand piano. We were sitting there wondering what we were going to do and she's playing away. There was that feeling that you couldn't do anything about it because it was a private hospital and we all knew her. So she played and eventually she stopped and walked out. Great characters. They'd been there for years. We all knew them and they all knew us and it was good fun in some ways.'*

Supervision on placements was improving, as has already been mentioned. The whole feel of the School in the 1970s seems to have been one of striving for more and more efficiency, whether in teaching, the curriculum, or selection of students. A student's experience on placement could obviously be very much affected by the quality of their supervision, and the courses introduced under Miss Van Garderen served to improve this. Also by 1975 all staff were taking part in visiting the students on their various placements. By the mid to late 70s a small number of mature students were joining the course and local placements were now reserved for them so they might stay with their families. Students re-sitting exams were also able to do a local placement to help them use the School's facilities for revision.

So, many changes were taking place on the academic side of the School, what kind of life were the students enjoying during the 1970s? Very early on in the decade more mature students were enrolling –

several in their mid 20s, two of whom had families. The 1978 Study reported that 10% of the overall intake was mature, but the number of male students was still very small, usually no more than one individual. One student from the mid 70s remembers the mixture of backgrounds as being quite varied. *'There were still those students who came from a fairly privileged background, who drifted into occupational therapy because they enjoyed the craft work side, and those who were really very keen to be occupational therapists.'*

The students do seem to have become more vocal since the 1960s. They had achieved quite a breakthrough in writing their long letter of complaint to Mr. Heritage in 1974 and were at last granted representation on the School Management Committee the following year. From putting in minor requests for a photocopier and transport to Nene College, by 1980 they were addressing major national issues such as requests that the course become a degree and that the Clearing House offer greater information on each School. Closer to home they asked for more time for private study, changes in teaching methods and revision of exam papers. It seems that some of them at least sought the greater independence of learning and research offered by a degree course. Staff on the other hand saw a conflict. They feared that in allowing students greater freedom they risked failing to get them through their exams.

In 1975 a new national uniform was introduced and on request Miss Van Garderen allowed the girls to abandon their stiff, starchy grey and red tunics and don the more modern style. In actual fact, the students in the early 70s had learnt to adapt their grey and red tunic quite successfully to the latest fashion: *'We all ordered our grey tunics in the shortest length possible (and decent) and then ordered the blue wool capes in the longest length. These, teamed with knee-high leather boots, we thought made the whole outfit acceptable.'* Miss Van Garderen was still very strict on her students' appearance, especially outside the School. *'If you were seen out in your cape and you had jeans on underneath, we would all know about it. VG would come in and say, "Somebody has reported a student down town wearing jeans and a college cape". It was not allowed.'*

During the 1970s the annual prize-giving and garden party event seems to have changed its character. By 1979 it was described as the Open Day and Prize-Giving, indicating a less formal approach to the proceedings – a sign of the times. In this change of atmosphere it is

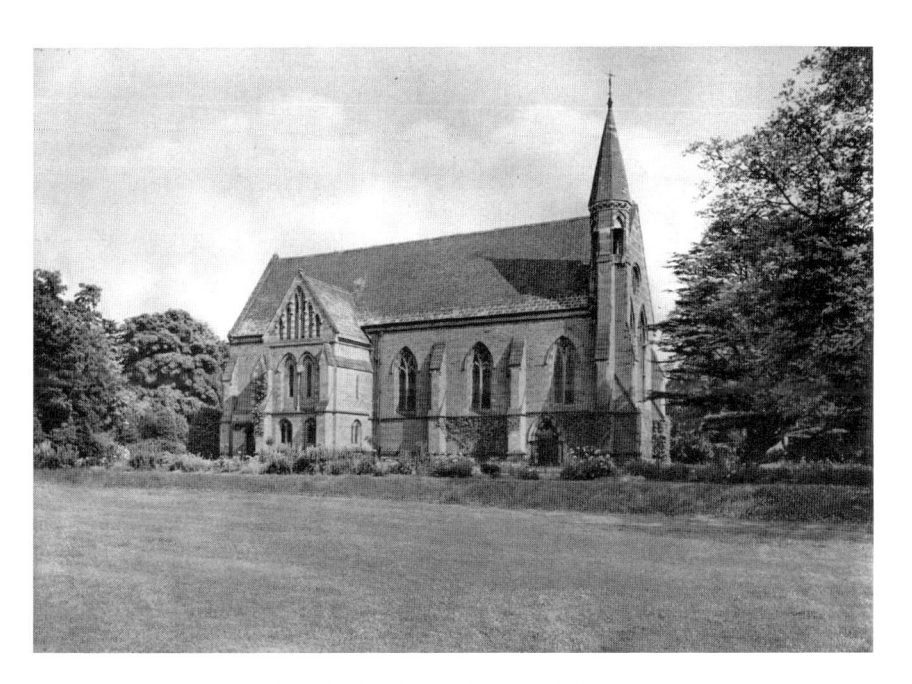

29. St. Andrew's Hospital Chapel

hardly surprising that the annual St. Andrew's ball along with the Eligibles book did not survive. The last one took place in 1973. The School Committee decided to give the students a grant of £25 'in lieu of their annual dance'. The following year the girls were organising their own dance in a local hotel, inviting whoever they wanted. The demise of the ball does not seem to have met with much regret: '*1973 was the last ball – you know, the system where they hired in these men ... We were all hanging out the windows of Lowood as the cars arrived with these chaps in who were horrendous. And we said, "Oh my god, where have they got these chaps from?" They'd come from the Conservative Club. There were a couple who were OK, but on the whole they were – you know – as you can imagine. But they were well turned out, nicely spoken, and it was a tradition.'*

The usual antics continued at Lowood, some sounding well organised, reminiscent of 'The Great Escape': '*There would be a sort of whistle system where somebody would inform the students that the warden was coming, and all the chaps would come out of the bedrooms and whiz down the back servants' staircase. We weren't allowed any boys in the rooms, except in the sitting room ... We had to try and climb in windows late at night. There was a change of lifestyle in the early 70s – students in general were given more freedom. We were mixing that old traditional girls' boarding school atmosphere with these changes in society.'*

As with the ball, the halls of residence did not survive the 1970s' demand for 'freedom'. Even when Miss Dallas was still Principal in 1972 some third years were politely informing her that they were going to find their own accommodation after their year out on clinical practice: *'We were duly summoned to her office and told that if that was our attitude the hostels would be closed down and all students would have to find their own rooms. Well, this was quite a knee-jerk reaction and not one we had expected. Short-term rentable accommodation in Northampton was not plentiful. The shock to the college was that six of us ended up renting two residential caravans on Billing Aquadrome for three months! It was a very quiet and happy place to study.'* It was quite a momentous occasion when the last students moved out of Lowood in 1976. It seems that pressure from the students to be free to find their own accommodation, coupled with the availability of room in St. Andrew's Staff Residence led to the decision to sell Lowood off. It had been used as a hostel ever since it had been purchased in 1950. Perhaps it was with relief that Miss Slater locked the door for the last time on a house now silent and empty.

Thirty five students were able to have single rooms in the staff residence. Even here they complained about the strictness of the rules. The rest had to find rented accommodation in town. No. 50 Billing Road was a useful addition to the hospital's properties as it was a Victorian four-storeyed terraced house close to the main gates, suitable as student flats. The girls could still not self-cater, using the hospital canteen for their two main meals, and being given a loaf a day, and every week half a pound of butter, a pot of jam and a slab of cheese for their breakfast. Some things did not change.

By 1981 Miss Van Garderen felt ready to retire. She was said to be quite a good age and to realise that the School now needed a younger person in charge. Although her replacement, Elizabeth Cracknell, saw much that was old-fashioned in the running of the School, VG had in fact introduced quite a few changes. She had worked hard to increase the number of teaching staff, even deciding to train them herself to avert the looming crisis. She had established a link with the new Nene College, tried hard to reduce the drop-out rate among her students, won approval for a new IAEM course in Psychology and Sociology, broadened the curriculum to include much more on the physical side with a programme of useful visits and external lectures, and begun work to improve the supervision of clinical practice. However, towards the end of her time as Principal, craft work was still seen as too dominant a part of the curriculum, being very wide ranging and lacking depth, and the students were still complaining about the concentration on lectures as the main teaching method, although a certain number of tutorials, visits and role-play situations were being used. Last but not least accommodation for the students had undergone quite a drastic change.

Looking at all these developments there is a real sense of how students' attitudes were changing – they were becoming more vociferous and independent. There is also a sense of the way in which the School along with the whole profession was striving to become more efficient. This was natural – as a new profession evolves, it must meet higher standards in order to establish itself. The assessment of physical disabilities, for instance, needed to become more scientific. The selection procedure of prospective students had to be made more effective and monitored. Above all occupational therapists began to think about the need to change the diploma into a degree.

In the beginning of this chapter it was mentioned that the 1970s were a decade of self-doubt for the profession. Schools of course had little time to worry about the definition or status of the profession as a whole. They were too busy training, encouraging and stimulating their enthusiastic students. Nevertheless, the discussions about the content of the curriculum reflect the uncertainty as to where occupational therapy was heading. Was there now an over-emphasis on the physical side? Was there not enough in-depth training in craft work? Was there just too much craft work? That is why this chapter has been called 'A Step too far?' Was the School losing sight of the psychiatric side of occupational therapy?

The final summary of the C.P.S.M.'s 'Study of Occupational Therapy Teaching Resources in the UK' in 1978 talked about the challenge of the danger facing the profession: *'Change is widely recognised as being necessary in order to reduce student wastage, to meet manpower demands and prepare students for a career which will require a continuation of learning and adaptation in order to meet the changing demands of medicine and society. This call for change should not be seen as a threat to those who have done much in establishing the profession and its training, but rather as an opportunity to capitalise on the enthusiasm and desire for co-operation and advancement which is very much in evidence.'* Changes were afoot in all places of occupational therapy education, not just at St. Andrew's.

The last word on the 1970s should go to one of Miss Van Garderen's students. Her summary of her memories about the School have the rather sad air of an era coming to a close: '*We thought St. Andrew's was one of the best. It had a nice air about it of being a traditional establishment with good values, and although we'd laugh about the uniform, it was something people felt was part of being a student. When we had visitors, all of us would rally together and make cakes and sandwiches. We just expected to do it. You'd stay behind and clear up and sort things out … We were a close-knit group in one building and we all rallied round and had some great fun. We were all young. It wasn't like today – it wasn't a case of having to get back home to the children. I think that atmosphere was a good atmosphere.*'

Chapter 7

'To wither on the vine'

Elizabeth Cracknell 1981 - 1995

Time of unrest and industrial action – Protests at cutbacks in NHS – Margaret Thatcher's Conservative government introduces market forces into the NHS and more privatisation – Increase in 'care in the community' - Call for 80% expansion of occupational therapy – Increase in marketing of profession.
Demographic change – Fall in birth rate in 1966 means decline in applications – Targeting of and rapid increase in number of mature students – 1989 Housing Act deregulates rent and leads to shortage of rooms.
Call for degree status – Staff expected to take degrees or Masters – Schools establish links with Higher Education institutions – Several new Schools founded – New Diploma '81 indistinguishable from a degree – New teaching methods to enable students to be adult learners – Concept of 'the reflective practitioner' - Schools have to compete for DHSS bursaries.

Elizabeth Cracknell took over from Maria Van Garderen in 1981. She was quite young compared to her predecessors and introduced a profound change in the atmosphere of the School, not only encouraging the staff to become more involved in its organisation but more importantly, enabling her students to become 'adult learners', responsible for their own education. She was part of the new wave of occupational therapists who saw the growing need to transform the therapy into a graduate profession. In 1985 the Council of Heads of Occupational Therapy Training Schools made a statement on the recent consultative document on the training for Professions Allied to Medicine (PAMs): *'During recent years occupational therapy has moved from a technician-based approach to a problem-solving one, and the work requires therapists to take a more consultative, professional position than previously. Courses have developed and altered vastly to accommodate these changes in role to the extent that there is now a mismatch between the status of the Diploma and the demands made on the diplomats who are required to take on high levels of responsibility immediately upon qualification.'*

To make the St. Andrew's diploma into a degree required establishing a firm link with an institute of higher education, and in Elizabeth's view this would not necessarily be Nene College. She gave herself eight years to achieve these two aims, not reckoning on the various difficulties that would hinder her in the process.

The general situation for occupational therapists was still promising as there was about a 20% shortfall in the numbers required. Care in the community was becoming more widespread and the number of frail or disabled elderly people was growing. In 1986, 1236 therapists were said to be needed to fill NHS vacancies, plus 1000 in local authorities. However, in 1985 severe cutbacks were introduced in the NHS which led to large protest demonstrations in various parts of the country. For the first time the profession was in evidence among the crowds. The Trade Union Council welcomed them on their first trade union event. The Chairman of the B.A.O.T. Council, Margaret Ellis, urged occupational therapists to respond to the Council's call for evidence on the effects of the NHS cutbacks. It may have been a slow process but a political militant spirit was beginning to develop in the profession.

In 1987 the government set up the Blom-Cooper Commission of Inquiry to study the future role of the occupational therapy profession with regard to demographic and social trends in the 21st century. The shortage was as a result of pressures such as the ageing population and changing perceptions of a patient's potential for rehabilitation. The Commission therefore recommended nothing less than an 80% expansion in the numbers qualifying by the year 2000. Other significant recommendations included the 'marketing' of occupational therapy and the consideration of a new name for the profession. It found occupational therapy 'something of a submerged profession' which was finding it difficult to eliminate an outdated image. It also saw a difficulty in maintaining an autonomous practice and suggested several reasons. Firstly, in the NHS occupational therapists were dominated by the medical profession and in Social Services, by social workers. This dependence meant it was difficult to allow market forces to prove the demand for their services. The outcomes of occupational therapy could not easily be measured and so the profession could be somewhat marginalised by the new managers of the NHS and Social Services, who were working on very tight budgets.

The B.A.O.T. and C.O.T. had made a very significant point in their report of 1986, The Way Ahead, in which they were to advise on the organisations' policy over the next ten years. In the light of the perception of how occupational therapy would be in the 21st century the writers of the report showed a great sense of vision: *'The use of activities should remain as an identifying feature of occupational therapy. Emphasis must be placed on the analysis of activity and its appropriate selection.'* They feared that if this was not done, the profession's identity might get confused. Other occupational therapy skills are also used by other professions, so the need was paramount to focus on what made the therapy unique. One former student remembers how difficult it was in her first post when she came face to face with this confusion of identity. *'Occupational therapists were not keeping abreast of the change and they were letting the use of adapted equipment outweigh the use of occupation as therapy. Often the equipment was used and the craft attached to it, discarded. Occupational therapy was becoming like physiotherapy. I remember being quite embarrassed as a young practitioner suggesting to a lady that she actually <u>weave</u> something while exercising her joints.'*

In the early 1980s Elizabeth Cracknell was not facing such momentous challenges. She needed to modernise her School. Making no major changes and altering very little in her first year, she knew that what she wanted to bring to the School would require a significant adjustment by the staff. She had trained at Dorset House and later married a Methodist minister. In 1962 they went out to East Nigeria with the Methodist Missionary Society, having to return five years later when East Nigeria declared its independence from the rest of the country and the threat of war loomed. With three young children, she took up part-time teaching at the Derby School of Occupational Therapy and then, in search of another challenge, took a degree in Social Psychology. The Principal of the Derby School invited her back to prepare a new Internally Assessed Externally Moderated Psychology course. Several years later Elizabeth felt ready to apply for the post of Director of Training at St. Andrew's School. During her interview she posed a question that took the panel somewhat by surprise: ' *"By what criteria would you consider me to be successful in this job?" "I think, Mrs. Cracknell, if it was a happy place, I would think you were succeeding" ... I think happiness is so important. If you're not happy, there's energy going on, anxieties, conflicts, tension. I thought it was a wonderful reply.'* She recalled her experiences at Dorset House in the 1950s and the strict authoritarian manner of the training – how she had been penalised for daring to question something Mary McDonald had said. The penalty involved having to continue wearing the uniform's probationary red belt for an extra six weeks before being allowed the students' green belt. She was going to run her School on totally different lines.

Despite the progress made by Maria Van Garderen, Elizabeth saw the School as still being set in the ways of the 1950s – *'It was Miss So and So, Miss So and So; students were not allowed to use the front stairs; there were staff loos and student loos. I took all the labels down. I did that in the first week. I introduced myself to the students by saying, "My name is Elizabeth Cracknell. My title is Mrs. Cracknell. You can use that with which you are most comfortable." '* One label which went up rather than down was at the entrance to the School. She realised with some surprise that there was in fact no sign announcing the existence of the School behind the hospital gates. The students clearly appreciated her changes. *'We no longer had to wear the student uniform in college and we were the first ones allowed to use the main stairs. So we were quite privileged.'*

The formal interaction between the staff at coffee time was replaced with a much more informal system. *'The staff came and had coffee with the Principal and sat in her room all in a straight line. We had maids who came and did things. It was so forced and false. I remember altering the layout of the furniture in the room because I didn't like it – to make it more comfortable. When I went back the next day the cleaners had been in and put it all back to where they'd had it before … I was very pleased that my first requisition from the hospital was a kettle so that the staff could make a drink when they wanted one instead of coming in and having a maid make one for them.'* A little kitchen was created upstairs and the timing of the mid-morning break made flexible. The upstairs bathroom was converted into a staff room where tutors could have more privacy to study and meet their students on a one-to-one basis. One of the old bedrooms was made into a student common room which was an unheard of privilege.

Changing the atmosphere of the School required more than these physical alterations: *'I tried to run it as a community, so I actually had community meetings to which most of the students came, but the staff found that too difficult. It was too early.'* Elizabeth's attitude to her students was radically new, for she saw them as her future colleagues. (One of the hospital governors, on the other hand, referred to them as 'children'.) Her innovation of a weekly staff meeting which initially looked at areas of responsibility proved a rewarding experience. *'It has been delightful to see the ways in which staff members have responded to the challenge of taking full responsibility for their own particular areas.'* Some staff were at first taken aback to find their Principal actually asking for their opinion.

Her relationship with her staff was developed through her introduction of the appraisal system. (Hers was the first department in the hospital to do this.) She saw her job *'to motivate the staff, change their attitudes, see what was necessary, keep them happy. I knew if the staff were happy, it would be fine. In the one-to-one appraisals I listened ... I feel it opened the channels. They were very wary of me when I arrived because it was just such a different regime.'*

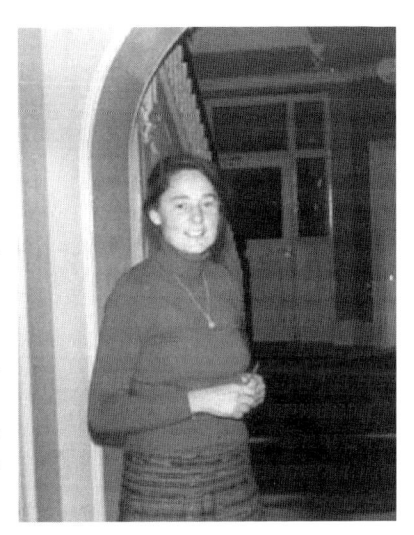

Elizabeth saw the small changes she was making as a way of bringing the School into the 1980s. Initially she did away with awards because they were divisive. The graduation ceremonies changed so that one year there was not even a dress code ('the jeans and chewing gum year'). The VIPs did not form a platform party but had to sit with the parents in the audience. In 1983 it became 'the Graduation Lunch'. Also, the students no longer had to wear their uniform in college – only on clinical practice. A photocopier was bought for Priory Cottage, even a computer for word processing, although the latter was said to be partly in an effort to keep up with the students, some of whom were already arriving with a fair degree of IT literacy. A Christmas party was held for the staff to celebrate the School's Golden Jubilee. Even the students were allowed to hold a party at Priory Cottage. Elizabeth took to explaining to them the feminist theory of why they were not part of a graduate profession: *'Universities used to have only male white Protestant students. They wouldn't take Catholics and women in years gone by. The women who started occupational therapy training in this country were pioneers – putting on a three year course for people outside the normal higher education system. They had battles to fight. They really were tremendous people – women doing things for women, which is why they wouldn't have men when they started. Men had somewhere to go – they could do various courses at university.'* Elizabeth's forthright manner was useful in encouraging support for the profession or in presenting the case for more funding, but it was not always well received: When Norman Fowler, Secretary of State for Health and Social Services, visited St. Andrew's, he apparently did not

30. *Elizabeth Cracknell 1984*

take kindly to her statement that *'rehabilitation is the Cinderella of the Health Service'.*

Only two years after Elizabeth's arrival a panel of inspectors noted her achievements in bringing the School up to date: *'Since September 1981 the total philosophy of the School has altered from that of a pragmatic training model to that of an educational model shared between staff and students in a more informal way. This has been a dramatic change for the staff who have not yet completely acclimatised themselves to the new style of management.'* This new style was even thought to have swung a little too far in the opposite direction – *'Within the new democracy a small measure of autocracy should be maintained, issuing some written instructions from time to time.'*

As far as the course was concerned, the School was always aiming at growth. Demand for places in the early 80s was high, five candidates for every place. The number of bursaries needed to increase before the intake could go up and Elizabeth sought funding outside of the normal DHSS channels – five private students were taken on quite early, and sponsorship was obtained in 1982 – five places from the Oxford Regional Health Authority and South Bedfordshire Health Authority. A prerequisite of growth was as always an increase in the number of staff. Some staff had started to leave during the 80s because they found that the pressure of going for degree status was not for them. It was expected that non-graduate members of staff would take a first degree or a Masters to meet the requirements of training a graduate profession. In fact by 1986 C.O.T. required that all staff in its Schools must take further study to equip them to teach a degree course. The number of staff under Elizabeth grew quite rapidly – achieving a ratio of 1:12 by 1983, which was considered acceptable. Two years later the staff's rate of pay moved at last from the Whitley (NHS) to the Burnham (lecturing) scale which helped to make appointments more attractive to prospective candidates. However, problems still remained. In order to attract clinicians into teaching at the School higher rates of pay had to be offered than prospective applicants were receiving on the Whitley scale. So new staff might be offered higher salaries than well established staff who had more experience in teaching. Elizabeth tried to rectify the situation by asking the hospital governors to grant pay rises to the existing School staff. Unfortunately, the governors saw this as setting an awkward precedent and would only allow salaries to be reviewed based on a revised job description.

Once staffing became adequate it was possible to devote more time to redesigning the curriculum in line with 'Diploma 81'. This was the radical new syllabus set by C.O.T. which updated the training and was in fact seen as indistinguishable from a degree. It enabled Schools to set their own exams, so courses became Internally Assessed and Externally Moderated (IAEM). Elizabeth relished the challenge presented by planning the School's own version of Diploma 81, finding it 'tiring but very stimulating', and by 1985 the School's course was validated by C.O.T.. One of the major practical differences was that it was taught over eleven

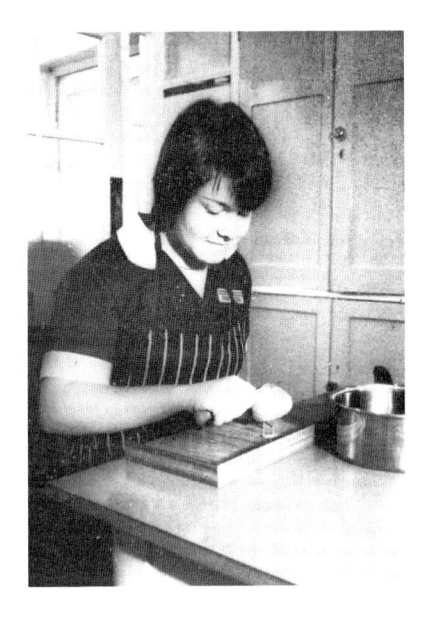

31. Learning to use an adapted tool to peel a potato 1984

terms – four ten week blocks, with clinical placements taking place for ten weeks each year. The syllabus followed 'The Life Cycle', with each term centred on a different stage: birth, infancy and childhood, adolescence, early adulthood, adulthood, mid life, and old age. This pattern of teaching served to reduce the mind/body dichotomy. Students were encouraged to take greater responsibility for their own learning, and more emphasis was placed on team teaching and assessments. For a few years it was complicated for the staff, who had to run two courses in parallel. Elizabeth resolutely refused to call the first group on Diploma 81 'guinea pigs'. They were given the far more positive description of 'pace-setters'. (The system of eleven terms only lasted a few years as it proved to be very tiring for the students and staff.)

Regarding the course one significant problem had come to Elizabeth's attention shortly after her arrival. It related to Anatomy and Physiology, which were being taught by Nene College tutors who did not have a paramedical background. When she went down to London to view her examination results in the summer of 1983, she received quite a shock: '*You knew what the national overall failure rate was, and I looked at mine and thought, "My goodness, we have over half the failures for Anatomy and Physiology"* ' *(*61% of the failures nationally). On all other subjects the results were excellent. She had had her suspicions about the tuition being provided ever since her students had told her that the skeleton in the corner of the classroom was never touched, except to insert a cigarette into its jaw. The solution seemed to be to employ an expert in the field who was more familiar with the requirements of a health profession. So an advertisement was placed for a tutor and Nene was given notice that their services on this particular part of the course would no longer be required. Dr. Janet Higgins was duly appointed and she revolutionised the teaching. A relatively large amount of money was spent on anatomical models and plastic bones, the hands-on experience helping the students to learn the details which they had found so difficult to grasp previously. Nevertheless, it is interesting to note that when the students were sent to Leicester Medical School to enhance their learning by examining corpses and seeing real muscles, the experience was not as edifying as might have been hoped. '*The muscles were very brown from the preserving techniques. We missed the colour coding which you get in the text books and the models!*'

Great efforts were also made to enhance the students' understanding of what life was like for disabled people. They were divided into groups, each with a particular aspect of disability to deal with. One group might have the problem of childcare. In this context it could be quite advantageous to have mature students on the course as one year was able to benefit from a student actually bringing in a two month old baby. Other groups might have to be blind for a day or confined to a wheelchair. One student recalls the day when the wheelchair group were given the task of going to Long Buckby on the train. Long Buckby station in those days (1992) was not wheelchair accessible and the railway staff made great efforts to help the group when they found themselves stranded at the station, unable to get across to the southbound platform. It was an amusing dilemma – should they be honest and reveal that it was only an experiment or should they see what solution the railway staff would come up with? In the end they chose the latter path and were allowed to go further north to Rugby where it was possible to change platforms. Their late return back to the School was forgiven. The day had been a useful learning experience.

One final point of interest about the curriculum – in 1987 Elizabeth reported that a third of the course was still being devoted to handcrafts. This seems quite surprising considering her enthusiasm for modernisation, but reflects the still prevalent attitude towards the importance of craftwork to occupation. However, the emphasis on creative group work meant that learning and teaching a craft was more an exercise in activity analysis and leading a group than finding out how to practise a craft with any great skill.

In general, teaching methods had been gradually changing during the 80s and the new ideas were written into the School's Diploma '81 course. No longer was it a case of lectures, a few tutorials and craft workshops; the methods were itemised under 'cognitive learning', 'skill learning' and 'personal growth' and included case study, discovery method, programmed learning, group work, role plays and discussions – apart from lectures and tutorials. The students look back on the innovative tuition with fond memories: '*We laugh now at some of the projects we had to do. We actually painted the common room – it was all to look at our interaction and working together.*'

Visits by external staff were also providing an enjoyable adjunct to the course, such as lectures on dance as therapy, sexual counselling and motorised wheelchairs. Commercial firms would bring in examples of the latter for the students to try out. The proximity of St. Andrew's was of course also useful to the students, who were able to learn about the particular fields of expertise being developed at the hospital on brain injury and eating disorders. A course was arranged on anger management which could be an important part of rehabilitation after a brain injury.

In the early 1980s clinical placements occupied the whole of the final year, some of them proving less satisfactory than others: '*I remember going to a London hospital and there were about 30 students from different colleges. You were just a number – literally. I was student no. 7. On my first day I went to the department and the woman there thought I was a patient and told me I was too early.*' The pressure of final exams in this year could be made worse by the need to travel back to Northampton. '*To do our final exams we had to travel up. I was coming from Norwich and had to take a train to Cambridge and then a bus. I've never had such a long double-decker bus ride! It stopped at every village. It took us forever to get to Northampton and we had an exam the next day.*'

During the 1980s however, work was being done to enhance the students' experience on clinical placement. The difficult economic climate in the NHS resulting in early discharge of acutely ill or physically disabled people meant that there was little time to treat these groups in general hospitals. It therefore became more important to choose clinical placements carefully to ensure students would gain maximum benefit from the experience. In 1987 the School decided to fund a full-time post of Clinical Tutor. Hazel Starmer was appointed and her work enabled a great deal to be achieved in this area. Although a Clinical Supervisors' Day had been in place for some years, Hazel started a monthly visiting day for the supervisors which proved very successful. By 1989 C.O.T. required work to be done on the idea of accrediting departments who wanted to take students. Hazel contributed to the pilot scheme within the Leicester district to put this process of approval on a surer foundation – a department had to reach a minimum standard in a number of specified criteria. Clinical practice constituted a third of the course; it was important to ensure its educational value.

Although Elizabeth had succeeded in tackling the various issues involved in modernising the School, there was one problem which could not be addressed so easily – demographic change. In 1966 the birth rate had started to fall, bringing with it the consequence of fewer school leavers applying for courses by the mid 1980s. The declining number of 18 year olds also meant that places even once offered were not so valued by the applicants, and St. Andrew's along with all the other Schools found that it could not rely on students to take up their place. In 1987 they were still interviewing candidates a week before term started. This decline was of course coupled with increasing competition from other Schools, some of whom had only recently opened, and some being already part of a university. During the 1980s the School had to be content with an average intake of 50 despite its ambitions to take on 60 or 70.

Various solutions presented themselves in the face of declining applications: to increase the level of advertising and to draw from a less traditional pool of possible candidates – mature people, both men and women. Elizabeth asked her new deputy, Annie Turner, to research how information on the School was being disseminated. The conclusion was that there was not much of the said information, and what there was did not travel very far. Most students had just heard about the School when they applied for an application form to go through the Clearing House system. So the School took various steps – updating a leaflet for libraries, career advisers and district occupational therapists, advertising in a careers directory for higher and further education and planning a promotional video. (These were apart from the usual measures such as open

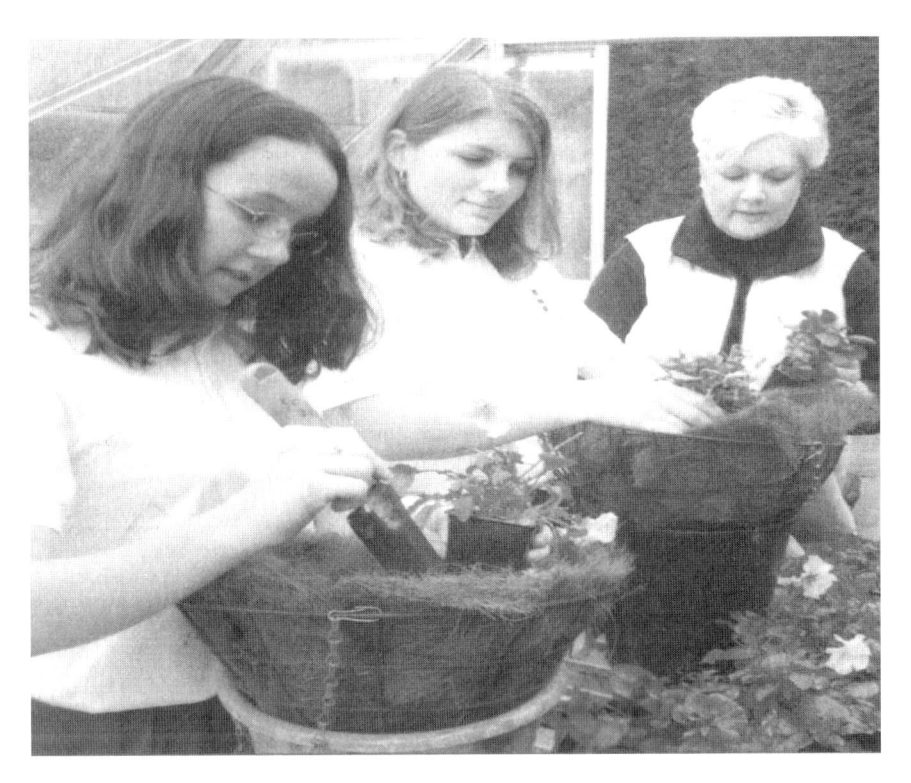

32. Learning to garden

days and updating the prospectus.) The video was produced by the Area Health Authority in 1990 and gave a vivid insight into the course. To illustrate the nature of occupational therapy short clips were included of students experiencing what it was like to bake a cake as a blind person, helping a client with an artificial leg to get dressed, and applying plaster on a splint. The various components of the course were also illustrated – anatomy and physiology, rehabilitation using a lathe and printing, the study of social skills in a group situation, the teaching of creative or leisure activities and drama, the enhancing of personal independence, the use of computer games to aid concentration, plus the more academic side of 'OT Principles and Practice' encompassing management, communication and research.

The publicity material laid emphasis on the valuable link with the hospital and stressed the suitability of occupational therapy as a career for older people whose maturity and life skills could prove useful in relating to clients. Previously it had been policy not to accept students from the local area, but now this was changed. Local people were actually targeted. An open evening was held for mature people, leading to much interest among those attending, although there was still a lack of male applicants.

One of the most significant solutions to the declining number of applications was the decision to further the process of changing the course into a degree programme. In 1988 Dorset House, the home of occupational therapy education in Oxford, was known to be linking up with Oxford Polytechnic in order to do just this. Students, especially mature ones, were likely to favour Schools where they could qualify as graduates. By 1989 Cardiff and St. Andrew's were the only Schools not to have developed close links with higher education. Which institute of higher education should St. Andrew's seek to join? Nene College was not the automatic choice. In 1984 Elizabeth had considered Leicester, Loughborough and Bedford. The arrival of the new Director of Nene College, Dr. Martin Gaskell, in 1989 was the catalyst that cemented the link with Northampton's own college of higher education. If the School became part of Nene, it would be beneficial to both sides. Occupational therapy enhanced Nene's portfolio of courses, for the college was already building up a significant range of HE health-related courses in chiropody, midwifery and nursing. Health-related courses formed a significant part of Nene's plans for future expansion. St. Andrew's would benefit from having a degree course supported by a local institution with all the practical advantages which this offered to its students.

A Statement of Commitment was signed between the two institutions in April 1990 when they agreed to work together to develop the Occupational Therapy course. Each would maintain their independence and integrity with separate governors and financial responsibilities. The School would remain part of St. Andrew's Hospital but submit its courses to the University and professional bodies, with Nene advising and cooperating on the development and teaching of its courses. A Joint Academic Advisory Board was set up to facilitate the collaboration. Almost immediately the decision was taken to prepare for the validation of a BSc in Occupational Therapy in 1991. It was a very demanding exercise to be undertaken in such a short time, but it was important that St. Andrew's competed with all the other Schools already offering a degree programme.

Great changes were therefore taking place academically and administratively. The students were still based at Priory Cottage most of the time, but they, like the staff, realised that times were changing. On a practical level, their meals at the hospital staff restaurant were no longer subsidised, (later they were not able to use it at all), and bus transport was laid on so that they could leave St. Andrew's at midday and be at Park campus for lectures at 1pm.

Looking back over the whole of the 1980s the student experience had been changing all along. Their very first encounter with St. Andrew's at the interview stage had been a different experience from the selection procedure in 1992. Elizabeth recalls how in the early 80s parents would often accompany their children to the School for the interview, and she would try to usher them into town to get them out of the way. Psychometric tests were still used, as In Maria Van Garderen's time. If you were found to be an introvert, it was doubtful that you would be accepted, although the results were always combined with what was learnt from your interview and the group discussion that assessed social interaction and leadership skills. Elizabeth encouraged the less mature candidates to take a gap year by offering them a place the following September. She recalls with some amusement the pressure that some fathers seemed to try to exert on Visiting Days: '*I found myself cornered in my room being drawn on "how to crack the selection procedure"!* ' By 1992 the procedure was quite different. Due to pressure of resources and lack of evidence of their necessity, individual interviews were no longer used. Applicants were selected on the basis of their application forms and references.

The proportion of mature students rose rapidly during the 80s – only 7 out of 47 (15%) in 1981, rising to double that proportion by 1992. Elizabeth had always favoured taking mature candidates: '*Northampton was known, and indeed Nene College too, for giving people a chance who probably wouldn't have a chance elsewhere. We did give people opportunities, particularly mums with children who felt they'd not had the chance of higher education.*' However, it was still difficult to attract men to the profession.

In 1981 first year students were living in the hospital nurses' home. 'It was run by someone like a prison warden who used to walk around in her hobnail boots, or so we said. The nurses' home wasn't very nice really. It was very bleak. We weren't allowed male visitors. The warden would walk along the corridors and knock on the door. We used to have pyjama parties to get round that.' Some girls had to live in rented accommodation. There must have been a shortage of local rooms because at least two girls remember having to cycle in from the villages of Nether Heyford and Cogenhoe – distances of about eight miles. Living so far out could be very isolating. By 1986 accommodation was no longer being provided by the hospital and the need was felt for a Hospital Accommodation Officer to negotiate with estate agents and landlords. The latter were reluctant to let out flats to individual students who only wanted accommodation for a few months between clinical placements, whereas they might be more willing to deal with a large organisation. In 1989 the new Housing Act deregulated rents, leading to a considerable rise in the price. Also, the rise in mortgage rates led to landlords selling off their properties, leaving students to face a shortage of flats and bedsits.

When St. Andrew's finally stopped organising the students' rooms in 1990, Nene College offered to take responsibility. In line with the separate finances of the two institutions the School would pay Nene a fee for their services. The YMCA on Cheyne Walk quite close to the hospital seemed a suitable building for Nene to lease as a student hostel. It was mainly occupied by first year occupational therapy students. On arrival they were disappointed, and their parents somewhat horrified, at the overall shabbiness of the place. Matters suddenly came to a head when Nene and the School learnt that the students had spoken to the press about their poor living conditions. A solicitor's letter had even arrived on the desk of Nene's Director. Inspection of the building revealed that the fire doors were all locked on the first floor, so it wasn't long before alternative arrangements were made. By 1992 there seemed a good number of convenient houses within walking distance of the School and the students were accommodated in these.

Those who started in 1992 were in the strange situation of having their first year almost totally at St. Andrew's and their remaining years were a transition period when they spent part of their time on the college campus. They recognised the advantages of having a better library and more access to computers, but *'it was difficult becoming anonymous, and the college felt very large. We missed the lovely grounds and felt neither one thing or the other.'* Instead of exams in St. Andrew's Great Hall they had to go to the Freemason's Hall on St. George's Avenue. Freemasons, not surprisingly, were not used to having ladies on the premises and there was only one ladies loo. Perhaps the streamers and balloons left over from a ball the night before went some way to enlivening the atmosphere.

1992 was also the year when the size of the intake went up considerably. There were now 65 students, of whom only about 20 were under 23. Of the rest there were about 20 under 30 and 25 over 30, the eldest being about 50. The 'boarding school' atmosphere of Lowood and the red and grey uniforms now seemed long gone.

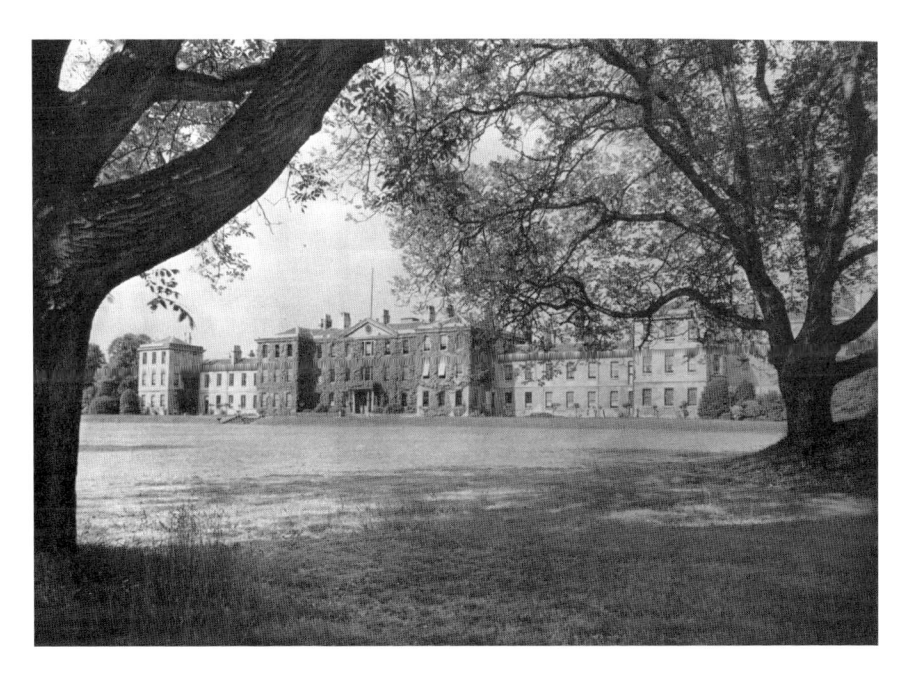

33. St. Andrew's Hospital main building

As the School and its students faced the changes brought about by joining Nene College and developing a degree course, another more dramatic change was being discussed by Mrs. Thatcher's Conservative government which would deal such a blow to St. Andrew's School it is hard to appreciate the effect it was to have on Elizabeth and her staff. It is the reason why this chapter has been called 'To wither on the vine'.

'Working paper 10, Education and Training' (EL (91) 24) was part of the White Paper, 'Working for Patients', which was published in 1990. The government sought to introduce the market economy into the training of the allied health professions. It therefore changed the funding system, taking bursaries away from the DHSS and giving NHS Regions the responsibility of allocating these bursaries as they saw fit. Regions were initially allowed so many bursaries according to the level of their population and not according to the number of Schools in their area. In 1990 Northampton was part of the Oxford region which was allocated 142 occupational therapy student bursaries. The South West was only granted 115, Merseyside, 70, both being less densely populated than other regions. Unfortunately the Oxford Region had two Schools and so

St. Andrew's would be competing with Dorset House for the 142 bursaries. The Region had been providing 20% of the qualified occupational therapists nationally and was now deemed to be 'an oversupplier'. To gain any more bursaries a School would have to market itself to other Regional Health Authorities and try to sell its training places. The idea was partly based on the assumption that students wanted to attend a local School in their Region and that they would subsequently take up work in that Region – as tends to happen in nurse education but historically not in the smaller professions. In this way Regional Health Authorities could fund their own occupational therapy workforce. The same system operated for physiotherapists and other allied health professions.

It is interesting to read how the DHSS tried to justify the new funding policy. It claimed that Regions were being encouraged to exercise choice and it was therefore appropriate that the ring fence round occupational therapy education be removed. Schools now had to operate in a way which would please provider units (i.e. hospitals and social services) – by offering good clinical placements and modular degrees, for example. A provider might require a module to fit a local need, such as a course on helping ethnic minorities. There was a wish for occupational therapists to come from a wider range of socio-economic backgrounds, so a School's selection procedure might need to change to take this into consideration.

To change from central to regional funding did not seem logical to Elizabeth. In actual fact Schools had always taken students from the whole of the UK, and on qualifying, students would work anywhere in the country. C.O.T. used this argument when opposing the change, stating that occupational therapy education was a national scheme and all schools ran on a national basis. The new funding had an important effect on the arrangements for clinical placements, as providers of placements had to offer them to the holders of the Region's bursaries. Thus, if St. Andrew's had a student who was not funded by an Oxford Region bursary, that student could not automatically go on a local placement which St. Andrew's had used in the past.

When information about the new policy arrived on Elizabeth's desk one morning in May 1990, she was so upset and shocked as she thought through the consequences, that she went home early to deal with the news in the privacy of her own home. She knew that the Oxford Region would favour Dorset House over St. Andrew's, the former being based in Oxford, the centre of the Region, and having had links with a college of higher education for a longer period of time than St. Andrew's.

It was fortunate that St. Andrew's had at least signed a Statement of Commitment with Nene the previous month and that their degree course was set to begin in 1991. In fact when Elizabeth subsequently talked to one of the NHS officers she learnt that they had hoped the St. Andrew's School would 'wither on the vine'. The Region was expected gradually to reduce the allocation of bursaries to St. Andrew's and allow it to close within a few years.

Once the shock of the new policy was over, Elizabeth wasted no time in fighting it or at least dealing with it as best she could. *'The concept to me of an internal market is a contradiction in terms, for according to the contracts I have seen, it is one which is managed and manipulated by the most powerful section of the organisation, and quality care of patients seems to be way down the line as everything seems to be run on an economic basis ... We are moving from solely an education service orientation to one which incorporates the world of business and the market economy, and we need to reframe our thinking to include 'provider', 'purchaser', 'budgets', 'tendering' and 'contracts'.'*

The whole debate about the effectiveness of occupational therapy, mentioned at the beginning of this chapter, now took on a new urgency. Employers of occupational therapists could influence a Region's policy on the number trained by the Region (and to be subsequently employed there). The Local Government Management Board, for example, were the people who influenced how many therapists were employed by Social Services. The whole profession, not just the individual Schools, needed to market itself to the relevant organisations. St. Andrew's was allocated 54 bursaries from the Oxford RHA in 1991, to be reduced to 33 in 1992. Fortunately, now that the course was a degree, students were eligible for LEA grants, although these were not as generous as NHS bursaries. In 1992 St. Andrew's won 17 bursaries from the Northern Region and Elizabeth set the School the target of attaining ten private overseas or sponsored students plus ten funded by their LEA.

New Schools began to be established, some radically different from the older ones. In East Anglia, for instance, a new School was set up in Norwich that combined the training of occupational therapists with physiotherapists. St. Andrew's was particularly affected by this new establishment because traditionally it had had a number of clinical placements in that area. These clinical departments would understandably now want to support the regional School they had helped to fund. It was a reflection on the well established reputation of St. Andrew's School that after the regionalisation of funding the number of applicants did not seem to go down. In 1992 300 people applied despite the loss of DHSS bursaries and the fact that the degree had still not been fully validated. (It was subsequently validated retrospectively, so students commencing in 1991 were able to qualify as graduates.)

It was clear, however, that the link with Nene College needed to progress, and in 1992 St. Andrew's School became part of the School of Health Science in the Faculty of Education, Health and Science. Elizabeth was now a Head of Department and the staff became employees of the College. The academic work would take place on Park Campus and the practical and clinical aspects at Priory Cottage. Priory Cottage was now leased to Nene for a seven year period and it was decided to retain the old name, which now became St. Andrew's School of Occupational Therapy (Nene College). It was thought that the association with St. Andrew's would help in recruitment and research provision.

Elizabeth was eager to point out all the advantages of the merger. The School was now able to draw on other staff to teach subjects such as Medical Sociology, Information Technology and Research Methods. Students could enjoy the Students' Union and all the various societies, and benefit from the Student Welfare Service. Financial matters were now administered centrally. The School's staff could enjoy the stimulation of teaching on other courses, such as movement studies, sharing ideas with new colleagues, and having the chance to submit bids for research projects. Nevertheless, Elizabeth's buoyant attitude hid the stress that she herself was experiencing. It was not easy suddenly to go from being Principal of a School to Head of Department, no longer able to refer to 'my staff' or exercise initiative freely and hold her own budget. The degree ceremony in 1993, for instance, was quite a momentous occasion as it was for the last cohort of students to qualify who had entered the School when it was still part of the hospital. Elizabeth even invited Elin Dallas and Maria Van Garderen to the event. However, she found that she should not have acted so independently; the School was now part of a larger institution and Heads of Department were not supposed to organise their own graduation ceremonies.

In the course of the next two years the Faculty of Education, Health and Science became the School of Health and Life Sciences and Priory Cottage had to change its name to Kelmarsh, following the pattern of naming campus buildings after local villages. Elizabeth's physical presence at Priory Cottage was very important in the coordination of the School's various activities prior to a final move up to Park Campus, and she remained in her office despite Nene's expectations that she would move up to the main campus. St. Andrew's was very sad to be losing the School. There was a sentimental attachment, but the governors understood the inevitability of the situation and that costs were just too great for things to continue as before.

Elizabeth was nearing retirement and she chose to go a couple of years sooner that might have been expected, for it was propitious to leave once the merger had settled down. She enjoyed being able to speak her mind in a more forthright manner once she had taken the decision to leave. '*I was retiring and leaving a super team to run the School. Once you know you're retiring, you can fight their battles – fight the battles for the course. You can do it more vehemently.*' As she prepared to leave in 1995 she started her staff off to do yet another five yearly revision of the course, assuring them that they were well equipped to do it now without her help.

One of her staff sums up part of her achievement: '*She changed the atmosphere of the School. She shifted it from being a place where you really didn't have a lot to say – you were taught, and this was how you behaved – more towards a very quiet disciplined process where students were adult learners. She shifted the dynamics significantly.*' Elizabeth herself was able to see the fruits of this particular change. She recalls a conversation with one of her finalists in 1992: '*It is a great joy to see how the finalists have developed throughout the three years. As one said to me today, 'I have learned most about myself'. This to me is the reward of being here. It is not just about helping patients develop their potential but students also.*' Subsequently, after her retirement Elizabeth was made an Honorary Fellow of the University of Northampton – a fitting recognition of her achievements in the field of Occupational Therapy Education.

On setting out on their new careers some of the students from this period remember how much they needed to draw on what they had learned during their time with Elizabeth Cracknell: '*When we qualified* (in the mid 80s) *we were forever trying to justify our role and what we were doing. Now, therapy as a whole is much more appreciated.*' The advent of multi-disciplinary teamwork in the 80s was another reason why it was becoming more difficult for outsiders to see what occupational therapy was all about. '*There was, and still is, a real blurring of roles because an occupational therapist might work with a social worker and they can both man the enquiry desk in a team.*'

Elizabeth had been faced with enormous challenges when she arrived at the School in 1981 – to change the School's diploma into a degree and to merge with an institute of higher education. As it happened an even greater challenge loomed when the changes in the funding system foresaw that the School might quietly 'wither on the vine'. That she overcame this problem and achieved so much in modernising the School reflects her great strength and leadership skills.

Final words on this chapter go to Elizabeth herself as in 1992 she reflected on the changes she had seen and the challenges she foresaw for the profession as a whole in future years: '*I was trained in the 1950s in the 'filling the empty jug' model or when on placement in the 'sitting next to Nellie' model. We have shifted from that model of training to an educational one which provides students with a much broader understanding of the context in which they work and the issues that arise, and includes investigative and evaluative skills required for the 'reflective practitioner' – the person who always questions and never accepts ... I went through the White Paper, 'Caring for People: community care in the next decade', and I was not happy with the overall thesis. Social Services are to provide 'care, practical help and support assessment of needs', but the word 'treat' is not in existence. I do not see the provision of aids and ergonomic adaptations as the essence of occupational therapy ... It is but a small aspect of the work. Clearly as a profession we are going to have to work hard to convince budget holders of the value of our service which can contribute so much to the quality of a person's life.*'

As the 21st century approached it seemed that the occupational therapy profession had survived the 1970s' 'decade of self-doubt' and was becoming much clearer and more balanced about its purpose, no longer concentrating on the physical side of the work to the virtual exclusion of the psychological. As the next chapters will show, this new sense of purpose drew on an interesting combination of viewpoints, one looking back to the profession's roots and the other moving yet further forward to unexpected and wider horizons.

Chapter 8

Moving On

Annie Turner 1995 – 2005

1997 Labour government elected – Advance of Internet and I.T. provision - 2000 government's new Strategy for Allied Health Professions calls for expansion and more funding - 2005 reorganisation of Strategic Health Authorities into larger regions.
Mid 1990s C.O.T. calls for emphasis on Occupation not Activity – Profession starts to return to original concepts behind occupational therapy in face of over-emphasis on 'Assess and Go' - Late 1990s craftwork virtually ends — 2002 C.O.T. rewrites syllabus, focusing on Occupation for Health – Increase in research - Early 2000s part-time and in-service study for BSc makes degree more accessible to mature students.

The new position statement issued by the C.O.T. in the mid 1990s demonstrates this period of looking back to the profession's roots. There is a new emphasis on the word 'Occupation' instead of 'Activity', which had taken pride of place since the 1960s. *'Occupational therapy enables a powerful need – occupation … The goal of occupational therapy is to promote people's health and well-being by enabling meaningful occupation. Occupational therapists believe that health can be influenced by occupation.'* The statement draws on the unspoken values and beliefs of societies as long ago as the period of the Ancient Greeks and the Middle Ages, as mentioned in Chapter One: *'Occupational Therapists seek the active involvement of people, empowering them to be participants and partners in improving their life-skills. This enables them to influence their own environment and to maintain and enhance their own health and opportunities. The partnership involves the understanding and creative use of the environment and resources; the person's abilities, skills and aspirations; and the occupational therapist's broadly based knowledge and experience.'*

It is an attitude which would have been recognised by Dr. Casson as she tried to motivate and inspire her clients in the 1920s and 30s. It was not the position understood by those doctors and medical staff who worked on the basis of the medical model. They saw medical intervention as the important factor in achieving success rather than working on the basis of the social model, which saw disability as the result of environmental restriction rather than restriction caused by shortcomings in an individual.

In 2000 the government seemed to be supporting the social model of disability when it published a new strategy recognising the importance of the Allied Health Professionals, 'Meeting the Challenge: a strategy for the AHPs'. More than 6,500 therapist posts were to be established plus new therapist consultant posts. This of course had an important effect on the existing Schools of Occupational Therapy, some of whom like Northampton were struggling in the face of a dwindling number of bursaries. Student numbers would have to increase dramatically in order to meet this challenge. In 2000 there were 21 universities and colleges offering Occupational Therapy degrees. In 2007 there are about 35. The new wave of funding will be discussed later in this chapter in as far as it affected the Northampton School.

The advent of information technology and the internet in the 1990s meant that the C.O.T. could also increase its networking activity. As part of the new encouragement of evidence-based practice the Clinical Audit Network Database was launched to enable more networking to take place related to research. As research became more and more established in the profession in the mid 1990s, the British Library started to publish research projects in the OT Index, an electronic database. By 2000 this had been replaced by the Thesis Collection on the C.O.T. website. Also, eleven specialist groups were developed in the College in order to further the study of the various areas of the profession which required particular skills, such as work with the elderly, people with learning disabilities, children, and work on orthotics and prosthetics, hand rehabilitation or remedial gardening. In 1997 the Research and Development Board and Group was established to lead on the strategy for the whole profession in the U.K., *'It was hailed as the start of a new era.'*

Of course the reform of the NHS mentioned in the previous chapter provides an important background to all these new developments. In the new world of the market place, targets and incentives, proving the value of occupational therapy was becoming ever more important to the status of the profession. The C.O.T. produced a leaflet entitled 'Who makes doctors better?' as part of its campaign to emphasise the value of occupational therapy in cost-effective primary care. It suggested how occupational therapists could help doctors achieve the new 'Health of the Nation' targets in areas such as chronic heart disease and stroke rehabilitation, mental illness, learning disability, sexual health, cancer care, and the enabling of safe discharge from hospital and independence for the elderly. On the other hand, in practice the pressures of time and finance meant that occupational therapists in community care were faced with the frustration of having their skills directed almost solely at assessment, home-visits and the supplying of equipment. Nevertheless the new 21st century saw a great burst of positive imaginative thinking on the part of the profession despite or perhaps because of the financial pressures of the new NHS market place.

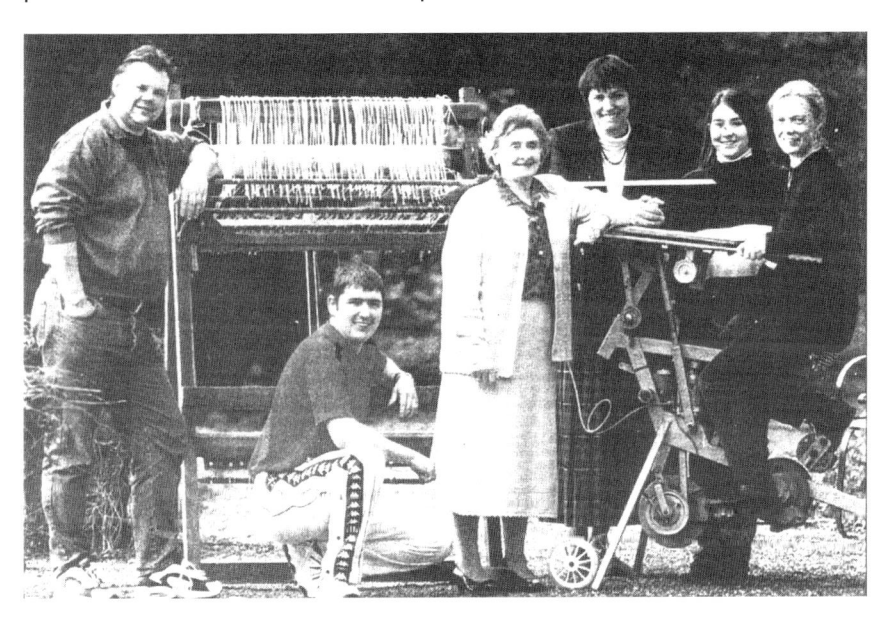

34. Moving out of Priory Cottage 1997
(reproduced by kind permission of the Northampton Chronicle & Echo)

Developments at the Northampton School reflected these two opposing trends. As the School eagerly moved its premises to join Nene College at Park campus and embraced the new syllabus, at the same time it had to forestall a potential disaster in 1996 when faced with the prospect of receiving no bursaries at all from the Oxford Regional Health Authority.

The new Principal, Annie Turner, took over from Elizabeth Cracknell in 1995. She had trained at Exeter and worked first in physical medicine, including a period overseas with VSO, before embarking on a teaching career at her former School. Her first post at St. Andrew's was as Course Leader in 1986, then as Principal Lecturer when Elizabeth retired and the School merged with Nene College. Annie's professional knowledge and expertise and strength of character played an important part in enabling the School to come through this difficult period and to draw on all the positive enthusiasm and excitement generated by this new call to 're-invent' the profession. *'When I came, the profession was very medically driven … What we did was to take on board a lot of new professional learning very quickly and then focus the programme with this new learning at the heart of it. So we became a school that had occupation as the professional drive for learning, as opposed to being based on the medical model with the occupational therapy bit stuck on the edge.'*

The School was particularly fortunate in having Annie to lead it because she was in fact at the forefront of the new thinking behind the profession, having written the first edition of a text book, 'Occupational Therapy for Physical Dysfunction', in 1981 and completing work on the fifth edition in 2001. It had soon become the standard book on the subject. She worked on the creation of the new C.O.T. syllabus at the turn of the century and so was able to ensure her School would be at the leading edge in professional thinking. In fact in 2000 she was awarded a Fellowship of the C.O.T. Subsequently in 2007 the University of Northampton awarded her the title of Professor of Occupational Therapy in recognition of the contribution she has made to her profession.

'When I became Head of Division, we had to find out what it was that we were good at, what would attract people to Northampton, what was it about us that would make people want to come to Northampton as opposed to any other School, given that Northampton, geographically, is a place people pass through. People don't know Northampton. It hasn't got the glories of Oxford. It hasn't got the big city appeal of Coventry. It hasn't got the beautiful geography of Exeter. We really had to stand back and say, "What is it about this place that is going to attract people to come?" So we made sure professionally we were leading edge. We introduced a philosophy for the whole School and the undergraduate training that was focused on the underpinning philosophy of the profession. That hadn't happened before.'

Before describing the changes that took place under Annie's leadership, it is important to reflect on the huge upheaval involved in moving the School out of Priory Cottage, away from the privileged environment of St. Andrew's Hospital. Being part of St. Andrew's meant more than the physical location. The School was a reflection of St. Andrew's charitable status which had a deep influence on the Hospital's activities, not only in setting up and subsidising its own occupational therapy school to provide students for this relatively new profession, but in opening its doors to NHS patients who could not easily be treated elsewhere. The Hospital always sought to remain at the forefront of psychiatric endeavour. In 1992 the Chairman of the Governors, Sir John Robinson, reported *'St. Andrew's is a charity, not a commercial organisation, though it operates in a commercial environment. Its success cannot be measured only financially, but also in terms of its contribution to the mental welfare of this country. Its role, therefore, includes seeking out those areas where there is distress as a result of unmet psychiatric or psychological need, and either to meet it or to direct policy-makers towards it; all this within the constraint of ensuring the Hospital itself remains financially healthy ... (St. Andrew's is committed) to the tradition of working with difficult to treat and treatment-resistant patients to enable them to lead lives which are as productive and satisfying as possible.'* In the 1990s the Hospital's work had expanded from dealing just with psychiatric illness to working with developmental disability and brain injury *'in a highly skilled, caring and therapeutic environment'.* Three quarters of its work today is still in support of the NHS.

It had always maintained a great interest in the School and was sad to lose it, although it realised that the time was right for a merger with a higher education institution. Since the mid 1960s two of the governors and the Administrative Officer had been on the School Management Committee. One of the governors, Mrs. Morgan, had chaired the committee in the beginning and she was succeeded by Lady Braye, who had been a governor since 1978 and had a great interest in education, having been a teacher herself. Lady Braye chaired the committee right up until the merger with Nene, when she was invited to be one of the college governors in order to achieve some degree of continuity. She was given responsibility for the School of Health and retired in 2005 after many years of service to occupational therapy education in Northampton. *'She maintained her role as our link governor, which was absolutely lovely ... She was hugely supportive ... She always felt quite positive about us.'* Lady Braye recalls the sadness of separating the School from the Hospital that had been responsible for its very existence. The governors always wanted to put back into the NHS what they were taking out, so although they were no longer able to subsidise the School itself, they provided a bursary and preferred clinical placements for Northampton's occupational therapy students. Also, the Chief Executive, Paddy O'Riordan, became a member of the College Court, and Dr. Martin Gaskell was made a governor at the Hospital, thus maintaining the link between the Hospital and the School.

Initially the School took the name of the St. Andrew's / Nene College School of Occupational Therapy and the governors asked that the new title should be clearly evident at the approach to the School. Sadly, when the final move took place in 1997 the name was changed. One of the students from this time has voiced her disappointment: *'We were angry at losing the name – they should have kept St. Andrew's in the title. St. Andrew's wouldn't mean anything to new students now. The School's history means so much – the name should have continued to show the connection.'* The move itself was difficult for those students who had enjoyed life at Priory Cottage. *'It was sad because it was so lovely and the building was like stepping back in time really. You could imagine lots of students passing through ... Even though Nene had a lot more facilities like a library on hand, we were sad to leave.'*

The sad farewell to the Hospital was marked on the 27th March 1998 by the ceremonial planting of an acacia tree on the lawn behind Priory Cottage. By September the Cottage itself had become the Lady Braye Centre – the location for St. Andrew's educational and training service. Also a few months previously in November 1997 over 250 former students and staff marked the occasion of the move with a gathering to bid farewell to St. Andrew's. It was here that the Friends of St. Andrew's School of Occupational Therapy was launched by Annie Turner and Beryl Warren, an esteemed 'old girl' known to many through her long career in occupational therapy and Chairmanship of Council of the C.O.T.

The Friends had two main aims – to act as a focus for past students and to support members and the School by providing a network of professional expertise. During the ten years of its existence the group has organised open days, dinners and reunions, publishing a popular annual newsletter and raising funds to provide prizes and awards for the current students. Years 1 and 2 have benefited from a book token prize for academic excellence and excellence in fieldwork respectively. 3rd years vote for the Student of the Year. In 2003 the first award was made to enable a student to attend the Occupational Therapy national conference, an event which always provides great inspiration for the student involved.

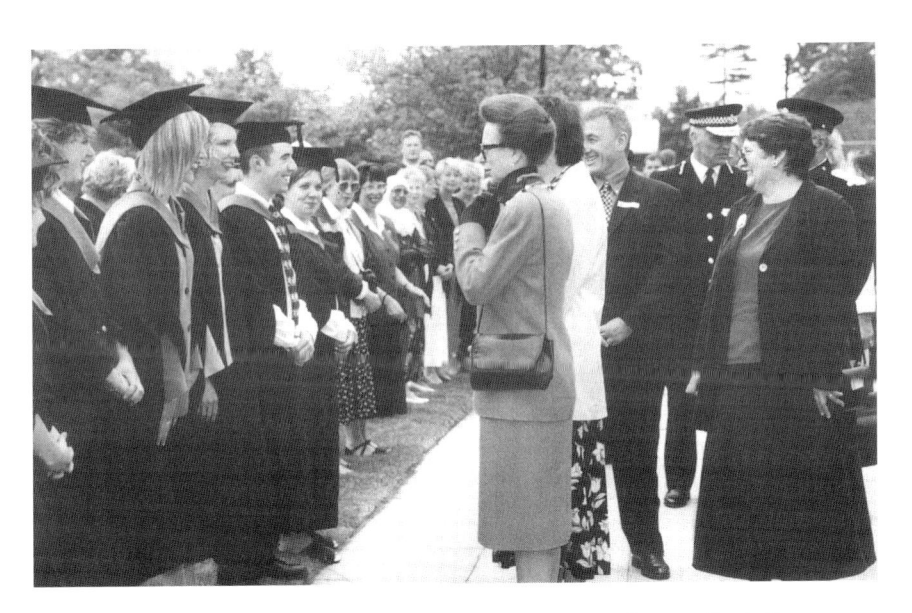

35. The Princess Royal opens the Kelmarsh building at Park Campus

The existence of 'The Friends' had been important when the School was searching for an identity on the occasion of the move away from its roots. It had been difficult to make it self-financing, however, and with the move, past students who had trained at St. Andrew's felt no affinity to Park Campus. The new students who have graduated from Nene (now the University of Northampton) have enjoyed feeling part of the whole college / university. It was felt appropriate therefore, in 2007 to merge the Friends with the University Alumni Association. At the final AGM it was recognised that time moves on. As a way of ensuring that the past would not be forgotten the Friends commissioned this book, jointly funded by St. Andrew's Hospital and the Division of Occupational Therapy at the university.

As the School marked the move away from its roots in all the usual ways, what was happening on the ground amid all the inevitable chaos of packing up and moving out? Clearing out the attics unearthed some gems of occupational therapy education – *'wrought iron work tools, boxes of embroidery silks, cooking pots big enough to feed an army, prototype bicycle fretsaws, treadle fretsaws, old examination papers, dusty books on leather tooling, knitting patterns, and loom, looms, looms!'*

The task of designing and building the new School on Park Campus was given to the architects, Gotch, Saunders and Surridge. One of the main features was to be a state of the art Activities of Daily Living

Suite comprising a kitchen, bedroom and bathroom. There was even to be a vegetable and sensory garden for rehabilitation where students could put their horticultural skills into practice. Annie wrote an article for St. Andrew's Hospital magazine and her words reflect great excitement at the sense of the end of one era and the beginning of a brand new one: *'Our brave new world? Purpose built and still smelling of paint our new building is situated in the heart of the campus. Being surrounded by libraries, IT services, healthcare colleagues and 10,000 students constantly reminds us that we are in the world of academia.'*

Staff and students were delighted to learn that the new School was to be officially opened by the Princess Royal. '*Students volunteered and staff organised. The grounds department worked flat out landscaping the building site, neatening the car park, laying turf, building gates and erecting lights – there is no doubt that if you want to get a thing finished, invite a royal visitor!*' As the Princess Royal toured the building she was treated to demonstrations of digging, weeding and watering in the garden as well as work being done in the ADL suite. Everyone appreciated the time she took to talk with them, especially the students, and they were impressed by her knowledge of occupational therapy.

So in 1998 the School was well and truly open for business, with the future seeming bright and promising. However, the legacy of Working Paper 10, issued back in 1990, was still in evidence. At the same time as she was planning the move out of Priory Cottage with such energy and enthusiasm, Annie was facing the fact in 1996 that the Oxford Regional Health Authority had now ceased to award the School any bursaries whatsoever. For that year all the students were funded by LEA grants and were therefore denied the advantage of having their fees paid and their maintenance grant take into account the cost of double rent during placements. Fortunately, however, the School was not about to 'wither on the vine'. The following year it received the good news that the Bedfordshire and Herts Health Authority was to award them 12 bursaries. Then four years later in 2001 this number went up to 60. Annie recollects that prior to the contract with Bedfordshire '*the School was struggling, and if it had gone on much longer we would not have survived ... Although the first contract was only very small, it gave us our self-esteem back and also meant that we were able to demonstrate we were able to attract funding, and it wasn't anything to do with standards. When we failed to get a contract, the word on the street understandably was that we weren't up to standard. But actually it wasn't standards, it was politics. That was a very difficult message.*'

During the late 90s, however, the intake remained high, being about 80 in some years, 60% of whom were mature and local, therefore attracted by the proximity of the School to their home. In 2000 a surprising drop in applicants nationwide meant that the intake went down to less than 60. Then at last, in 2000, as mentioned in the beginning of this chapter, the NHS Plan announced major reforms and investment. It was calculated that there was a 40% shortfall of occupational therapists and so there was an urgent need for more schools and training places. The market economy had not proved so effective after all. The government recognised there was no point in investing in building new schools when one school was under capacity. Some schools were not even recruiting to their number of bursaries, so the money was not being taken up. Northampton, on the other hand, found it easy to recruit even though it only had 13 funded places in its cohort (12 from Beds & Herts and one from St. Andrew's). The government therefore awarded the School a 'national contract' and Annie remembers the satisfaction of being able to announce ' *"We are a national School with national placements"* ... *That gave us our first sense of stability.'*

Being a 'national' school with 'national' placements was not as easy as it sounded, for the Oxford and Coventry Schools still claimed the clinical placements in Northamptonshire, being the regional schools for the county. The situation was so difficult that Annie was in fact in despair. She had, however, a very good placement team who succeeded in finding fieldwork all over the country. The School was reaping the benefits of having put a great deal of work into this: *'We were one of the first schools that put a lot of resource and energy into practice placement. What had happened in the past was that although a third of the training is on practice, it never had a third of the resources in terms of staff. We did a lot of research about practice learning and assessment and we all did an enormous amount of PR work with our partners because we had no contracts. The only way we got placements really was begging or through the old girls' network and by offering students who were good students. We kept our standards up. We made sure our students knew what they were doing while they were there. We assessed them well. If people were having troubles we went out and supported them. So we put a lot of energy into the external working of the School. We still do that. That is still a big part of the heritage of that time.'* So the School's reputation was good and getting better. *'People told us, "Your students are so well supported; your assessment is good; you have well prepared students."'* As has been seen in previous decades, strong leadership and the hard work of its staff helped the School to weather the storm and move forward in professional and educational terms.

After 2002, when the School had no less than 75 bursaries, another reform of the NHS led to changes in the structure of the Regions. The Leicestershire Northamptonshire and Rutland (LNR) Workforce Development Confederation was formed in 2004, and at the same time Bedfordshire joined up with Hertfordshire. Having no other rivals in the LNR Region, it was no surprise that the School received 20 bursaries. 60 bursaries still came from Beds & Herts. In 2006 the NHS was again re-organised, this time into much larger regions, including the East Midlands and the East of England Strategic Health Authorities. LNR went into the former and Beds & Herts into the latter. The School felt fortunate in having commissions from more than one Region; funding looked far more secure, and placements opened up in both the East Midlands and the East of England. As Annie has said, *'Now (2004) we have about 100 bursaries; to me that smacks of stability – financial and political stability.'* The effect of the problems of the previous decade remains to a certain extent: *'It did have an effect on the way the School developed, because I feel that in developmental terms we're about five years behind where I'd like us to be. We had to have all our energies focused internally – just on survival really ... In the halcyon days we used to get about ten applicants to every place. At the very lowest ebb we hardly had one applicant to a place. So it had a huge effect. But we did manage to nearly fill, and we did survive, and we did manage to attract people – mostly local people. At the point when we had so few bursaries we did a survey and 90% of prospective students who didn't accept offers said they really liked what they saw but couldn't afford to come. So we knew the issues were not about our division or about our standards. Our problems stemmed from politics. '*

One difficulty that was linked with the sudden rises and possible subsequent cutbacks was staffing levels. Prior to 2005 there had been about 10 – 12 staff, but this figure had to go up dramatically to 20, of whom half are part-time. It is an interesting reflection on the changes that have taken place since the 1990s and before, that staff are now expected to have or be working towards a masters level qualification. All are occupational therapists. One of the current staff who remembers the 1970s explains how few qualified occupational therapists there used to be on the staff; *'There was a cookery teacher with a qualification in home economics; a lady with a background in art who did a lot of the basket weaving and woodwork, and there was an art teacher. For lectures we'd have doctors and physiotherapists come in to teach anatomy, physiology, psychology, sociology – those sorts of things.'*

As has been seen, the beginning of Annie's period as Head of Division was affected by the excitement of the move to Park campus and the difficulties incurred over funding and placements. What other changes took place under her leadership? In connection with the staffing issue she would like to put more energy into post-registration education, because of the effect this has on the local practice community. The range of courses

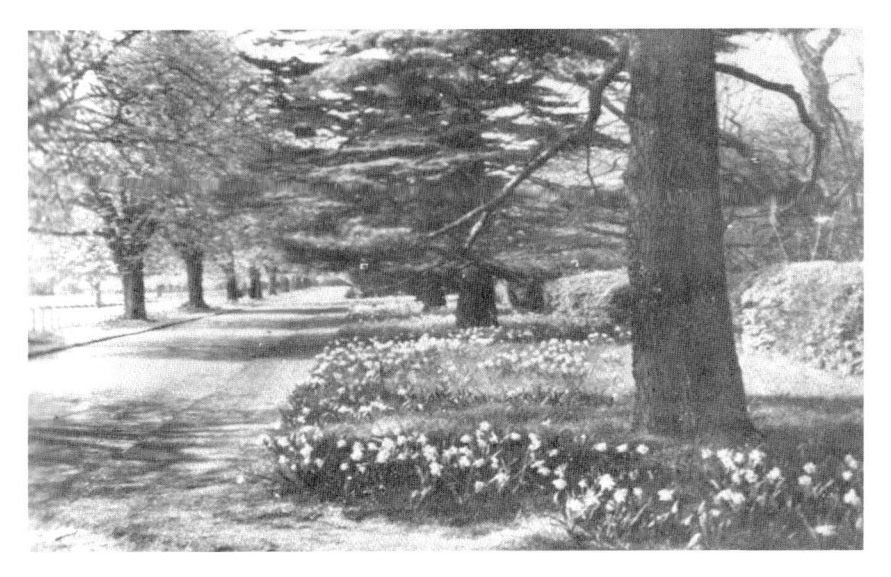

36. The avenue in St. Andrew's grounds

and types of degree currently provided in 2007 is wide compared with how it was in the previous decades – a Foundation degree is planned, a full-time, part-time and in-service BSc in Occupational Therapy. A BSc in Occupational Science, is being explored, and an MSc in Advanced Occupational Therapy, and Continuing Professional Development, including the C.O.T.'s Accreditation of Practice Placement Educators' Scheme, are also part of the Division's portfolio.

The task of running and organising the School has therefore grown enormously. In 2005 the job of Head of Division was divided between two people: Sue Griffiths took over the new Principal Lecturer / Divisional Lead post with responsibility for the organisation of the School, while Annie became responsible for external links in order to generate income. She works two days a week with the Open University developing the Foundation degree for Health and Social Care, one day a week on the Health Professions Council, which is responsible for maintaining standards within the health care professions. The other two days of the week she is the external link, meeting with local occupational therapy managers, the professional body, other Heads of School, for instance, and is responsible for the development of the post-registration portfolio.

Sue Griffiths has been associated on various occasions with the School since the 1980s and was in fact a student of Elizabeth Cracknell at Derby. She became involved in curriculum development alongside her career as a clinician in mental and physical health settings and wrote, for example, some short post-registration courses to be run at Nene College.

In 2000, a few years prior to this leadership reorganisation Annie took the bold step of appointing a Reader to the School. This is a senior academic post that leads on research activity such as bids for funding, disseminating research results at conferences and publishing articles. What made the post unique in 2000 was that the Reader would also become involved at undergraduate level. There was only one Occupational Therapy Reader in the country – at Oxford Brookes, who concentrated solely on research. Northampton's Reader actually impacted on the teaching. *'That was something we were very proud of'*, says Annie. Dr. Susan Corr qualified in Dublin and worked in Cardiff as a clinician before entering research and education. Her work in Northampton has been of enormous importance in enhancing the quality of the undergraduate research. In most other Schools research is confined to literature reviews that require a student to compile a comprehensive list of research papers on a particular topic, but Susan's energies have allowed Northampton's undergraduate occupational therapists to continue with primary research within the restrictive confines of the Department of Health's Research Governance guidelines.

One of Susan's major achievements at the School is to launch the Health Through Occupation Research Group (HETOC). The formal launch took place in September 2006 at the 5th Occupational Therapy UK and Ireland Symposium, hosted by the University of Northampton and attended by delegates from Sweden, Chile, Australia, the USA and Ireland. There are four key themes in the planned research for the group: Older People as Occupational Beings –which involves 1st year students as data collectors and for which there is a collaborating partner, the University of Jonkoping in Sweden, who are replicating the study; Well-being and the Quality of Life, for which, for example, one member of staff is working on in a study of the perceptions of individuals with neurological conditions recently discharged from a rehabilitation institution in Italy. The third theme is Occupational-based Occupational Therapy which includes research to further develop the Morriston Occupational Therapy Outcome Measure (MOTOM), and finally, Arts and Health. For this latter topic 3rd years as well as a Masters student have been looking at creative activities as treatment. In 2007 Susan secured the appointment of the Division's first Visiting Fellow, Dr. Mike Lowis, a psychologist, who has an active role in the research activities of HETOC, in particular the older people as occupational beings project.

Susan reflects on her contribution to the Division: *'In terms of research, as a profession we're in our infancy, but I think what we're doing here is that I've built up a foundation and a culture where research is now much more part of the psyche of everybody. There's much more drive to do it and there are practical activities going on that facilitate novice researchers to be part of this. The Older People project is very useful because students can not only collect data but use it if they choose the topic for their dissertation.'*

Her involvement with international collaborations and think tanks serves to put the School well and truly on the map. In 2007 she attended, for example, the 2nd International Think Tank on Occupational Science in the USA where work was carried out on setting up an international society for occupational science. Also one of her areas of expertise is 'Q methodology', having used it in her own PhD studies. This has aroused considerable interest and it is thought she was the first in the whole profession to publish research using it. It draws on qualitative and quantitative approaches to research and is designed to achieve as scientifically accurate a picture of people's opinions as possible, being based on a framework of statements which are sorted within a pre-defined parameter. In a similar scientific vein, Susan was involved in the development of MOTOM, a precise tool to measure the outcome of occupational therapy treatment and one which is clearly of great value in light of the drive to prove the clinical effectiveness of all health service treatments.

It is clear that Annie, Sue and Susan now preside over a vibrant school at the forefront of occupational therapy education and research – something which Annie would freely admit she feared would never happen in the dark days of the late 90s.

Chapter 9

Looking Forward

Sue Griffiths and Annie Turner 2005 –

2006 many occupational therapy posts frozen leading to job shortages - 2006 new Foundation degrees to train up Occupational Therapy Assistants – Modular system makes degree more accessible to mature students - 2007 all Schools re-focus on Occupation for Health as core philosophy - 2008 new BSc in Occupational Science of interest in the new re-focusing of the profession.

The funding, staff and research activity are of course a vital part of the background to the School in the new millennium, but it is also interesting to consider the content and structure of the current degree course and how different it is from the course offered in earlier years. At the end of Chapter 7 it was suggested that the profession had started to look back to its roots; this was to have a profound effect on the way in which students were trained. In 2002 the C.O.T. undertook a radical re-writing of the syllabus. Annie was involved with this work which led the profession back to focus on 'Occupation for Health' – the prime motivation behind early occupational therapy.

'The syllabus completely changed its focus. Its hub is now about knowledge of people as occupational beings and what happens when people cannot meet their occupational needs. So philosophically it's just turned on its head ... Our professional roots got rather smothered in the mid and late 20th century because with the establishment of the NHS, occupational therapy went into the health service. Because the NHS is dominated by doctors and nurses, occupational therapy became subsumed within the medical model ... (The new focus still expects) occupational therapy to analyse and use activity, so it's always surrounded by 'doing'. We do a lot of practical stuff, but the professional focus has changed.' It is now based around the premise that occupation is a health agent. *'We have an ADL room here, but it's sparse compared*

to what we had in the early 80s. Then, students spent a lot of time actually practising techniques – hoisting somebody, getting somebody into a wheelchair, walking – we would spend hours learning how to walk up and downstairs. All that's virtually gone. Students are expected to do that on practice.'

The re-focusing of the syllabus has meant that the Northampton School has been able to make 'Occupation for Health' the core module; Anatomy, Physiology, Psychology and Medical Sciences are now 'contributory disciplines'. However, the focus has now changed for all schools with the revision of the C.O.T. syllabus.

The emphasis on craftwork seems to have come very definitely to an end. *'We don't do craft. That's all to do with the history of the profession ... a legacy from the Art and Craft movement that was still permeating through into the 50s and 60s. Now what drives professionals is occupational science. As a culture in this country handcraft is not what people spend their time doing ... We do get some very creative students but also those who are creative in a different way – in their thinking or their actions.'*

The Reader, Dr. Susan Corr, has made some interesting observations on the importance of studying Occupation as opposed to learning how to teach craftwork: *'I don't have a problem with any activity being used to help an individual. What I do have difficulty with is making people do an activity. "Why should I do weaving? I've never done it before; I've no interest in it. What will I gain from it?" (Occupational therapy) should be about enabling an individual to tap into an activity that they enjoy. (Having said that, when you go to Scandinavian countries, the crafts that they do! They're not sitting in front of the television 20 hours a week or whatever. They do things.) I don't think occupational therapy departments should be filled with looms; neither do I think they should be filled with computers, but I think there should be a wide range of activities. Let people experience different things, because they don't know until they sample them whether they might like them or not. I don't think more crafts should be taught, anymore that we should teach more computer games. What else do people do? – They go to the cinema, eat out, cook. I just hope the students realise that the menu of occupations for every individual can be really varied. Unless they appreciate how very different people's interests can be, they won't understand how to best treat somebody.'*

The rewriting and revalidation of the degree course which took place in 2002 is a regular process to ensure that the content and structure is up-to-date and in compliance with any intervening legislation, professional knowledge and regulations affecting the students' education. A look at Northampton's list of modules helps give an insight into how the focus of the training has changed:

- Occupation for Health, defined as the study of healthy living within an individual's unique environment. Practical components include activity analysis and the therapeutic use of occupation.
- Contributory disciplines – Psychology, Sociology, Biological Sciences, Social Policy, as they inform occupational therapy thinking and practice.
- Tools for Professional Practice – for example, personal learning styles, manual handling and the use of assistive technology.
- Professional Context – the concept of professionalism and expectations within the health and social care context.
- Clinical Reasoning, through enquiry based learning – the study of case scenarios to enable the student to assess, plan and evaluate intervention.
- Professional Practice – clinical placements in a variety of settings. These involve 8 weeks in the Spring term of Year 1, 10 weeks in the Autumn term of Year 2 and 12 weeks in the final Summer term.
- Research Methods – In the final year a student completes a dissertation of 12,000 words.

As has been mentioned already, the majority of students are mature (defined now as over 21). Annie makes an interesting observation on the way the older students may react differently to the 'new' focus of the course: *'The programme has a psycho-social base and teaches how the values that you hold underpin your interaction with other people. (The value base we teach) stems from the moral treatment of mental patients in the 17th and 18th centuries … I think the mature students find it easier through life experience actually to stand back and look at people as people. Some of the youngsters can find that quite difficult - having said that, they are adaptable. They are very much more cosmopolitan so they are very much more used to looking at people from different ethnic groups as equitable. So to look at people with enduring health difficulties … they have much more open minds about difference. Some of the mature students can find the equity bit a little more difficult, as opposed to the "I want to care for these people" bit.'*

As far as the module on Research Methods is concerned, on her arrival in 2000 Susan Corr developed a strategy to enhance the quality of undergraduate research, creating a list of topics which students could choose from which was based on the interests of the staff, for she was

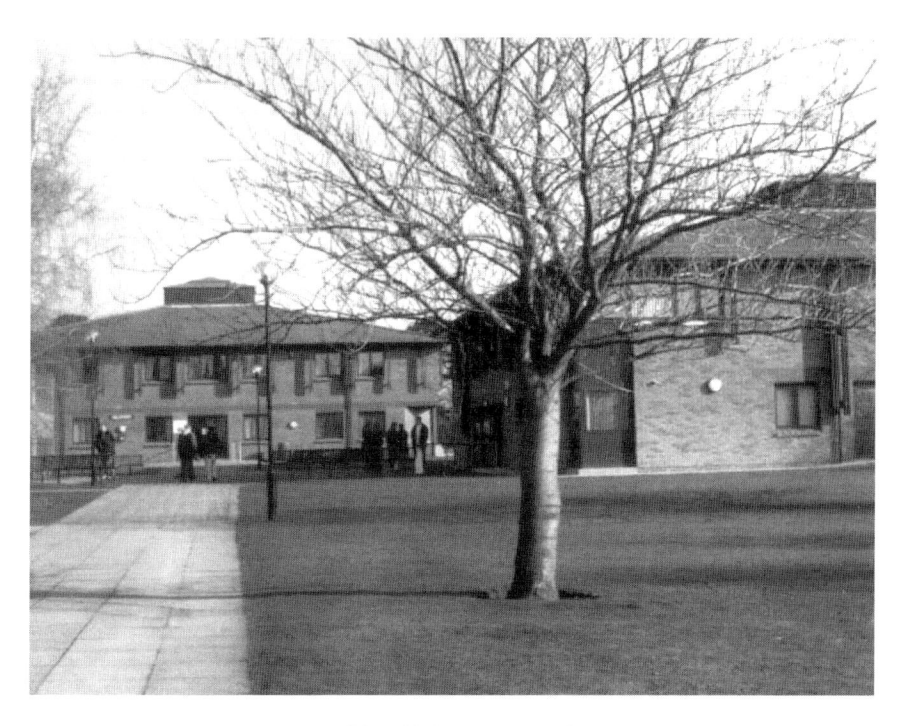

37. The Kelmarsh building

very conscious of the need to increase the amount of research being done by members of staff. One major obstacle to research in the health service has been the Research Governance Framework which was introduced in about 2001 and was based on the Helsinki international agreement designed to protect patients from being exploited. It imposed very strict conditions on the way in which health research could be carried out. As a consequence of the strict conditions many university departments decided not to allow their students to do primary research. Susan does not lay claim to being the sole inspiration behind Northampton's novel approach to the problem; several staff have supported her in this. Nevertheless, it was an exciting breakthrough when the Division realised a way round the issue of research governance. The students would carry out research on people who were not patients, but who were of interest because of their engagement in occupations, whether they have a physical or mental condition or not. Annie sees this initiative as a reflection of the way in which the Division had to learn to overcome problems in the difficult time of the late 90s. '*It is a sideways step round the system, which is what we learnt when our back was to the wall – How do we get round this system and not be smothered by it? ... What we've done is look at the science that underpins occupational therapy, which is Occupational Science, and students are able to gather information about people's occupational performance. They can do that on healthy people; they can do that on disabled people who are no longer actively receiving NHS care.*'

Susan explains how it works: '*Our students have done things like interview para-Olympic sailors. They were being interviewed for their experience of sailing – nothing to do with their clinical care. We've accessed participants in poetry writing groups and asked them questions related to their experience of writing poetry, not their experience of health care. Any questions related to health would be on the impact of the activity on their health. In some cases an interview might be too sensitive, so we'd do questionnaires. Students have accessed people in the community attending an eating disorder group, but it was felt that it would be more appropriate to ask the participants to fill in a questionnaire and a time-use diary. So we've established clear boundaries to ensure that primary research can be conducted on selected groups of people, the focus of which is about the relationship between their engagement in occupations and their health, but not their experience of the health service.*'

With Susan's support students have been able to write up their research into papers to submit for publication or present at national and international conferences. It is of course a great inspiration to have this opportunity available. Several former students with Susan have published their research in journals, including one on the impact of strokes in the workplace in the British Journal of Occupational Therapy, and another one on occupational changes in first time motherhood in the Journal of Occupational Science. One former student gave her paper at the College of Occupational Therapy conference and won the award for Best Presentation by a Novice Practitioner, while others have presented their research at the annual conference of the Irish Association of Occupational Therapists and at an international Q methodology conference in Norway. The staff too have benefited from Susan's support, two having become authors for the first time, with papers published in peer-reviewed journals; several have presented at national and international conferences, and Judith Knight became the Division's first PhD student in 2006. The undergraduates' experience of research is invaluable preparation for the world of work. One of the former students who graduated in 1995 has explained how most of her career has involved research in some form or other, such as service reviews, service development, or efficacy of treatment.

As far as the structure of the course is concerned, it reflects the current trend for flexibility. There is no longer one set way of studying for a degree in occupational therapy or one source of funding. There were three routes in 2006 – full-time (over 3 years), part-time (3 days a week over 4 years), and in-service (a secondment to allow part-time study coupled with part-time employment as an occupational therapy support worker). Unfortunately the in-service route will not recruit from 2007 because places on this route are not being commissioned.

The part-time route can be equally hard, with students juggling roles as parent, carer and/or employee alongside their work at the university. However, it has been amazing to see how successful some of the part-time students have in fact been, the most remarkable being the student who broke from her studies to have a baby, returned briefly before breaking again to have another baby, and then finally returned to graduate with a first-class honours in 2003.

All the part-timers tend to be mature students. For them life can seem quite daunting with the expectation of being one older person among lots of 18 year olds, but as one student has said: *'When I first enrolled I was wondering how old everybody would be, and when I walked into the classroom on the first day I realised I was not the oldest one – there were ladies in their fifties - and it was lovely because it gave a balance. I think life experience is good, and I think when people have a lot of life experience it brings another dimension to the work. You are able to empathise with people on a different level.'* For this same student, entering the occupational therapy profession was a particularly rewarding experience, for when she made her first enquiries she was a mother of two young children, searching round for a career now that she was no longer married. *'Whether it was people changing career or coming to a point in their lives when they were wondering what they were doing ... I knew as soon as I came to the Open Day this could be a job I really wanted to do for the rest of my life.'*

Mixing study with family life is not easy: *'Family need to be supportive as well, as there are times when you need to be very focused. I think you need to be honest with yourself and admit that sometimes you do need to take a break. You are not Superwoman, (well, not all the time anyway!)'*

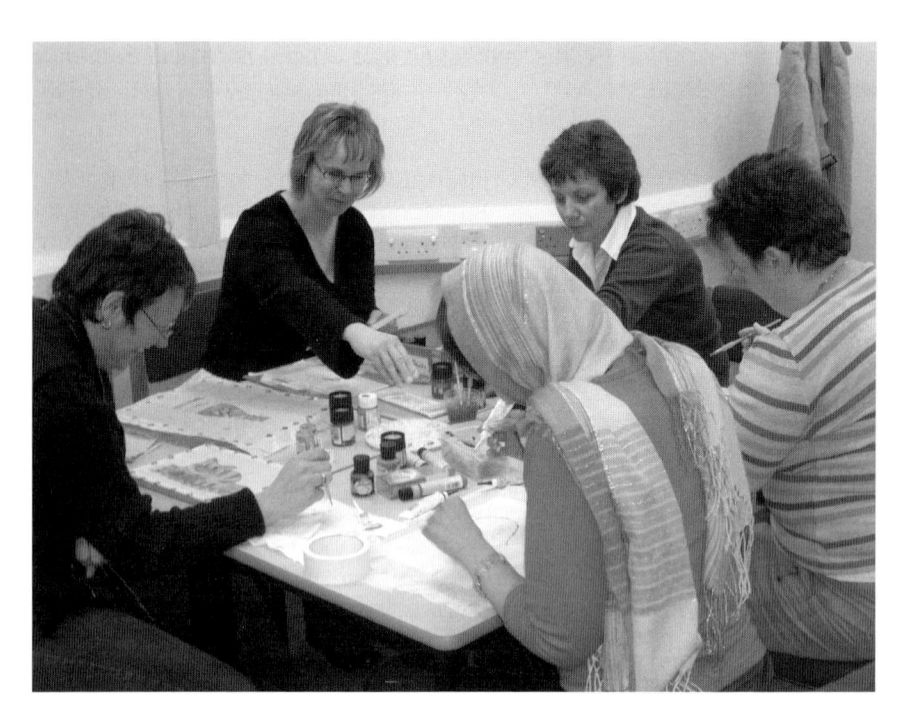

38. Learning silkscreen painting 2007

Wisely some of the mature students with other commitments do not set their sights unreasonably high. *'I was just after a "mum's degree", as they called it. We just wanted to pass. I just wanted 40% on my essays. I didn't care if I got 60% or 40% as long as I passed.'* Some, perhaps younger students set themselves very high standards. One of the tutors recalls *'When I trained (in the 70s) you either got a diploma or you didn't, whereas now students are very aware of their ability and what degree classification they want to come out with. They put themselves under a lot of pressure.'*

Of course there is also added financial pressure as grants have not kept up with inflation: *'When I look back to when I trained in the 70s, I was given a full LEA grant. It was tough being a student, but finances weren't a particular issue. Students now, to get themselves through university, are having to take on part-time jobs at evenings and weekends. That's a big issue. I feel they are under more stress – a lot more stress. There are a lot more services around to support them. You've got the university counselling services and GPs on site. We've got personal tutors. We now cater for more students with special needs. In my day if you got stuck with something it was Olive, the School Secretary and Everybody's Mum. Olive would sort you out. Students are under a lot more pressure.'*

In a way it is strange but significant that student life in the 21st century should seem beset with more pressures and difficulties than sixty years ago when post-war life seemed so lacking in comfort and convenience. Tutors have also talked of the difficulties that some students now find in mastering the academic skills: *'One thing students find hard to do now is put an essay together because of different teaching methods at school. GCSE papers can be short questions and answers, so the whole process of putting an essay together is quite a challenge.'* IT skills may also need to be honed because students need to type their essays and use Powerpoint for their group presentations.

The method of assessment is now coursework and seen exam papers and may seem easier compared to the reliance on exams in previous decades, but this kind of assessment can in itself be a pressure. One student who graduated in 2002 recollects: *'The finals almost finished me off. We were given two papers at the same time, one written and one for the viva; then a third paper. We were only allowed to take in 150 words of notes to the written exams to jog our memory. We had a choice of three questions and two weeks to prepare.'* A world away from learning by heart the bones, muscles and nerves so that you could recite them with your friends over breakfast.

The introduction of modules has had a favourable impact on the educational experience. Students must pass each of the six modules each year in order to progress. It has the advantage of enabling a 'Step on, Step off' system whereby they can leave after Level 1 if necessary and gain a Certificate in Health and Social Studies, or after Level 2 to gain a Diploma in Health and Social Care. When circumstances prove more favourable, a student can return to the degree course to carry on, but only as long as they can 'show currency', i.e. show that they have been practising, caring or working in a voluntary capacity in the meantime.

The number of compulsory modules has meant a lack of options in the course, and this arrangement is also being changed in order to move with the times. Sue Griffiths comments: *'Options are a good thing in education and excellent as an occupational therapist because we're all about facilitating people's choices and empowering them to do what they want to do. We have to be a bit cautious in order to maintain professional standards, but we are thinking of including modules from the School of Health such as in Sport and Exercise, Nursing and Social Work. We may even include the Volunteering module.'*

So the whole structure of the course has changed along with the content, bringing with it a depth and variety of study that is richer than ever before. The teaching methods have also been developed to keep up with the new thinking and new demands and are regularly assessed for their effectiveness. *'The trend in higher education within Health is for people to be much older and not go away from home as much. We need to respond to that change by delivering the programme in a way that allows as many people as possible to access it. So it is useful to deliver a couple of modules as distance-learning so that people can study it (at home) … Everything is posted on the internet. We no longer have piles of handouts at great cost that students file away and never look at.'* Students have also pointed out the value of the Northampton Integrated Learning Environment, NILE – an email system which enables students to access one another without even coming on campus. There are therefore plans to expand the facilities for 'work-based learning', 'distance learning' and 'e-based learning'. Annie sees the changes as part of the drive to change the paternalistic culture of adult education. The teaching approach is certainly much more scientific, efficient and consumer-orientated.

'Problem-based learning' is one example of the modern style which is seen by some to have advantages as well as disadvantages. One former student from the 90s has commented on the new style of occupational therapist who has been trained using this method – *'Problem-based students are good at finding out information, but don't have the grounding. I had a first year student on practice who mistook a lady with rheumatoid arthritis in her hands for a lady with a stroke – she hadn't studied the symptoms on her course.'*

There are two other types of course being planned as well as the BSc itself – the new Foundation degree in Health and Social Care and the new BSc in Occupational Science. The former will be administered by the School of Health, and the Division of Occupational Therapy will deliver some modules that will be accessible to Foundation students (as well as forming part of the BSc course).

It is clear that the recent development of occupational therapy education has been inspired by the drive for effectiveness, consumer satisfaction and a raising of standards in general, whether it be in terms

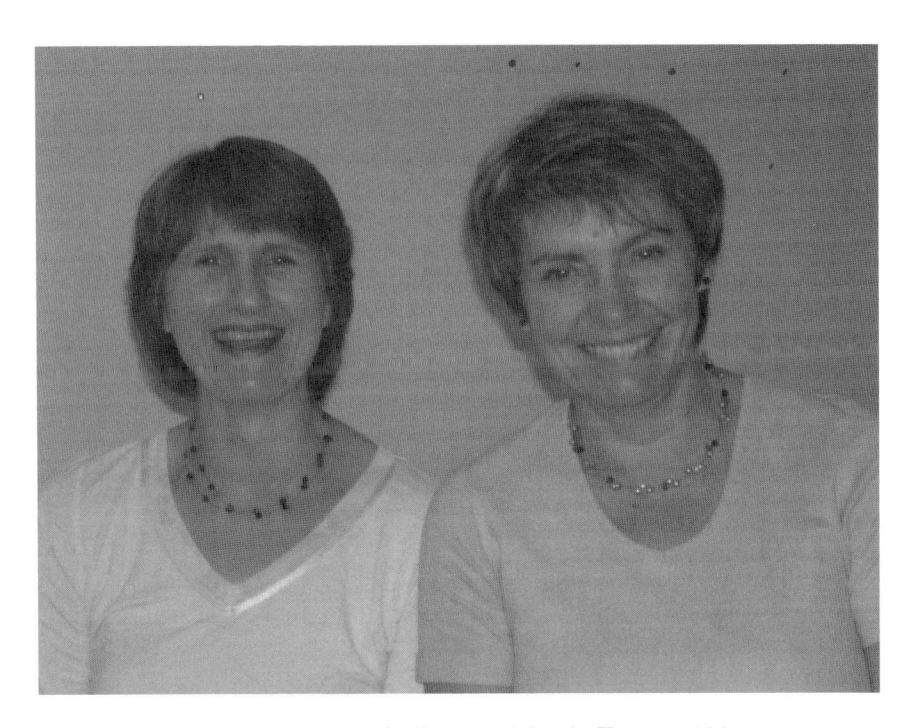

39. Sue Griffiths and Annie Turner 2007

of training up unqualified staff via the Foundation degree, regularly assessing 'learning outcomes' or providing optional modules. The supervision of clinical placements has also been the focus of a lot of hard work on the part of the staff to improve not only the quality of the training but also the variety of the work. The provision of training courses on clinical supervision has already been described. The timing of the placements themselves has also been improved. One of the tutors comments: *'When I trained in the 70s we went out for a year. We did a bit of theory; we did a bit of placement; we did a bit more theory; we went out for a whole year, and then we came back and did our finals. Now students do a block every year, so they're in, they're out, they're in, they're out, they're in, they're out. It's more of an integrated process. They are building on their theoretical base and trying to implement the theory in practice. It's quite a challenge for the students because they're always on the move. "Tools teaching" we call it – giving them the practical tools for working on the job – actual physical tools and also tools for verbal and written communication.'*

Recent cutbacks in the NHS have had an interesting effect on the type of fieldwork now being offered. At the end of Chapter 7 it was suggested that the profession's new sense of purpose draws on a combination of viewpoints, one looking back to the profession's roots and the other moving yet further forward to unexpected and wider horizons. It is these 'unexpected and wider horizons' which are relevant here. Annie has explained how in a poor job market occupational therapists need to free themselves and use lateral thinking to see how their skills can be used in non-traditional occupational therapy jobs. So now placements too are available in non-traditional areas - in for example, a local holistic centre that uses colour therapy as one of its means of treatment, a local residential centre for autistic people, the Motor Neurone Disease Association (whose headquarters is in Northampton), and Aquarius, which is a centre providing help and support for addicts.

Related to this lateral thinking is the 'New Ways of Working Day' that is now organised for third years. Here the students have the opportunity to find out about the variety of work available in the voluntary and private sectors as opposed to NHS work or Social Services work in the community. 'Condition Management Programmes' in the voluntary sector help people with mental health problems to find work. Workbridge, for example, works closely with the Job Centre and Volunteer Centre to enable such people to get back to work. One former student is now working for Motability, a voluntary organisation which enables physically disabled people to have their own transport. She has reflected on how in her student days in the early 90s there was no mention of the possibility of working for a charity. *'Work would be in the NHS or Social Services.'* Schemes like the local Spencer Project help people who are homeless and unemployed by enabling them to renovate a house that will become their home. In the private sector there is scope for work with brain injured people living at home, and in industry the National Farmers Union, for example, employs an occupational therapist to help rehabilitate agricultural workers who have suffered injury. Work can also be found in the prison service or in special education.

Great excitement has been generated over this kind of vocational rehabilitation and the scope it offers for occupational therapists to place themselves in jobs that would not previously have been suggested to them. This excitement is natural as this new area of work links so well with the roots of the profession in rehabilitation through occupation. It is a sad fact, however, that it is also a useful way to survive in the current world of cutbacks: in 2002 it was easy for graduates to find jobs. In 2006 only 75% were able to do so. In 2004 many NHS posts were frozen. Sue Griffiths has made the interesting observation that in actual fact the current job crisis could be liberating. '*Many community and hospital occupational therapists now find their work is dominated by the Health and Safety agenda of assessing patients to ensure that when they go home they are safe, dressed, bathed and fed. This agenda is called 'Assess and Go'. Occupational therapists would be better used to see how people use their time – they need to focus on what's really important: occupation.*'

One former student remembers being told by a doctor back in the 1950s that occupational therapists were some of the best lateral thinkers he knew : '*You need lateral thinking to be an OT*'. He was referring to their ability to adapt items to help people who were physically disabled in some way. It could be that this very quality of lateral thinking serves occupational therapists in more ways than one – helping them to find ways in which to return to their roots and use occupation as a means of treatment.

Conclusion

This book has been the story of a training school for occupational therapy, but it has also inevitably touched on the history of the whole profession and the wider social context. For those familiar with the development of occupational therapy it has hopefully encapsulated that history by telling the story of one particular school. For those who only experienced the profession in the decades after the Second World War it has perhaps shed light on some dramatic changes. It has hopefully given a picture of where the profession began, how it has changed, and where it is now.

There are some striking images within the story of the School that serve to illustrate what these changes have meant – early images of the students helping to alleviate the boredom of TB patients with the fur from old RAF jackets; using their wits and ingenuity to create a means for someone with a hand injury to open a door; or counting in the knitting needles used by a group of mental health patients. Images of the 1970s and the new demands for Equal Rights for the Disabled, of mental health patients being able to live in the community again, and now the 'Assess and Go' agenda offering a quick and safe discharge from hospital.

There is the sequence of events, reports and statements showing how occupational therapists have grappled with an identity crisis – the labelling of the 1960s as a 'watershed decade' for the profession, of the 1970s as the 'decade of self-doubt', then the C.O.T.'s reaction with their report 'The Way Ahead' stressing the need to focus on 'Activity', and the position statement in the 1990s calling for the profession to advocate 'meaningful Occupation'.

Of more relevance to the School's graduates there is the memory of the ease with which students in the first few decades could find their first job, the drastic experiment by the government in 1990 to allow market forces to determine the number of student places, then the NHS Plan of 2000 recognising the need to meet the shortfall of posts, and now the freezing of many of these and the need to move into non-traditional places of work.

There are evocative images of the course itself – ranging from students learning their bones and muscles by rote in the 1950s, to them now seeing their exam papers two weeks in advance. From young 18 year olds thrown in at the deep end caring for the mentally ill, to them now being carefully supervised on accredited clinical placements. The agonising over the meticulous standards of craftsmanship required in the 1950s, to the new talk of letting service users follow their own aspirations. A lecturer eccentric enough to write on the back of the blackboard, to staff earnestly assessing the effectiveness of their teaching methods. Interviews and 'What does your father do?' to 'How can we broaden the ethnic mix of our students?' Staff resigning in the 1980s rather than study for a degree, to an exciting combination of staff with Masters, Doctorates and even a Professor.

Then there are the images of the students' social lives – from 'Woe betide the students who got married' to proud talk of the 'mums' degree'. The stiff and starchy grey and red uniform, jazzed up in the 60s as a mini-skirt with knee-length boots and long cape, transformed now into practical green trousers and soft polo shirt. The strict close-knit world of Lowood and Rheinfelden, now replaced by mixed halls of residence where an occupational therapy student may be one among hundreds from other disciplines. The Ball and the Eligibles' Book, to the mini-rebellion in the 1970s and the 'jeans and chewing gum year' of the 1980s. The life of the staff too: Maria Van Garderen's formal coffee breaks in her office and Elizabeth Cracknell's triumphant purchase of a kettle.

In the background is the paternalistic image of St. Andrew's, giving grants to its needy students and appreciating the girls' contribution to the patients' social activities; followed by Elin Dallas' despair at this 'waste of time' in the face of the demands of the new four yearly inspections. The first tentative link with Nene College in 1970 that blossomed twenty years later into a merger and the move out of the idyllic hospital grounds. And now the full-blown world of academia with all its financial, social and academic pressures.

Apart from the images, there is the idealism that lay behind Mabel Thompson and Joyce Hombersley's rallying words in the 1940s – Mabel's quote from 1919: 'Restoration is at least as much a matter of spirit as of body', and Joyce's fervent call for research 'if we are not to slip back twenty years and find ourselves damned once more with the 'arty-crafty' label'. This idealism does not seem out of place in the Division of Occupational Therapy today. Building on its success in the face of considerable adversity, the Division can justly claim to be 'leading edge', with a culture and philosophy determined to look back to its roots and at the same time move forward to unexpected and wider horizons.

BIBLIOGRAPHY

Of interest in more than one chapter

Fogg, A. & Trick K. *St. Andrew's Hospital: The First 150 Years (1838 - 1988)* (Cambridge: Granta Edition, 1989)
Wilcock, Ann *Occupation for Health Vol. 2: A Journey from Prescription to Self Health* (London: B.A.O.T. & C.O.T., 2002)
Ayres, Henrietta *A Changing Community: St.Crispin Hospital 1876 – 1976* (Northampton: Northamptonshire Area Health Authority)

Chapter 1

Anon *Editorial* (Jnl A.O.T., Winter 1944-5, 21)
Archer L., M. Hutchings, A. Ross *Higher Education and Social Class: issues of exclusion and inclusion* (London: Routledge Falmer, 2003)
Argles, Michael *Technical and Scientific Education since 1851* (London: Longmans, 1964)
Assoc. of Occupational Therapists (A.O.T.) *Promotional Leaflet on OT* (1951)
Board of Control *Memorandum on Occupational therapy for Mental Patients, ref. 37051* (London: HMSO, 1933)
Bunyard, Janet *The correlation of the massage department with occupational therapy* (Jnl A.O.T., Winter 1940, 12)
House of Commons, Education, Science and Arts Committee Session 1955-6: *Student awards: memoranda* (London: HMSO, 1986)
Hombersley, Joyce *Letter* (Jnl A.O.T., Winter 1944-5, 21, 10-11)
Rogers, Byron *St. Andrew's Hospital* (Saga, June 1998, 62-7)
St. Andrew's Hospital *Annual reports*
Thompson, Mabel *Letter* (Jnl A.O.T., 1946, 26, 5-6)
Turner A., M.Foster & S.Johnson *Occupational Therapy and Physical Dysfunction: Principles, Skills and Practice*, 5th ed., chapter 1 (Edinburgh: Churchill Livingstone, 2002)
Wilcock A. & B. Steeden *Elizabeth Casson OBE MD DPM 1881-1954* (London: C.O.T., 2004)
Student contributions Pauline Barnes (Pickford) 1941-3, Rosemary Vaughan (Elmer) '41-3

Chapter 2

Anon	*St. Andrew's School of Occupational Therapy* (Jnl A.O.T., July 1948, 26-8)
Anon	*Obituary for Joyce Hombersley* (BJOT, Nov 1987, 50, 11)
A.O.T.	*Pre-training Educational Standard Requirements* (Sept 1951)
A.O.T.	*Promotional leaflet on occupational therapy* (1951)
A.O.T.	*Syllabus and regulations for the diploma* (1945)
Ministry of Labour and National Service	*Leaflet on occupational therapy* (ca. 1945)
St. Andrew's Hospital	*Annual reports 1944 – 57*
St. Andrew's School of Occupational Therapy	*Prospectus* (ca. 1946)
St. Andrew's School of Occupational Therapy Friends	*Newsletters* (1999, 2004)
Warren, Beryl	*Joyce Hombersley Book Fund* (BJOT, Aug 1988, 51, 8)
Student contributions	Joan Blesset (Dexter) '51-54, Anne Dickens (Ridgeway) '44-47, Pam Greaves (Davenport) '54-57, Brenda Mawby (Bullard) '55-58, Beryl Warren (Allingham) '53-56, Mary Watson (Baldwin) '51-54

Chapter 3

Castle, Phyllis	*Phyllis: Memoirs of a Misfit* (Bradford-on-Avon: ELSP, 2003)
Hombersley, Joyce	*Psychiatric training of OTs: speech to PMPA meeting at Northampton* (July 1952)
Hombersley, Joyce	*Speech at St. Andrew's School Reunion* (ca. 1978)
St. Andrew's Hospital	*Annual reports 1944-57*
St. Andrew's Hospital	*Obituary for Neville Parsons Jones* (Insight, Spring 1990)
St. Andrew's School of Occupational Therapy Friends	*Newsletter* (2004)
Student contributions	Sally Book (Holford) '56-59, Joan Bradley (Longson) '56-59, Pat Jebson (Fripp) '53-56, Barbara Jeyes (Bishop) '48-51, Susan Parker (Tennent) '52-55, Heather Powell '59-62, Audrey

Silkin (Bennett) '53-56, Hazel Starmer (Paige) '54-57, Wendy Valentine (Wilson) '50-53

Chapters 4 & 5

Anon	*Pink Bunnies and Baskets* (editorial) (OT, 1964, 27, 1, 1)
A.O.T.	*Lecture notes on occupational therapy for nurses in general hospitals and mental hospitals* (ca. 1950s)
Dallas, Elin	*Speech at graduation ceremony* (1993)
Heron, Alastair	*Occupational therapists and evaluative research* (SJOT, Mar 1962, 5-8)
Minto, Kate	*Speech at Joyce Hombersley Dinner, St. Andrew's Hospital* (1999)
St. Andrew's Hospital	*Annual reports 1957 – 71*
St. Andrew's School of Occupational Therapy	*Archives 1958 – 71*
St. Andrew's School of Occupational Therapy Friends	*Newsletter* (2002)
Student contributions	Barbara Beard (Manship) '58-61, Joan Bradley (Longson) '56-59, Anne Dickens (Ridgway) '44-47, Sheila George '66-69, Pat Jebson (Fripp) '53-56, Anne Lambley (Rutherford) '69-72, Pauline Leach '60-63, Brenda Mawby (Bullard) '55-58, Hope Mayne (Rickard) '64-67, Philip Ndekwe '64-67, Hazel Starmer (Paige) '54-57, Anne Strudwicke (Smith) '58-61, Sue Terry (Barker) '64-67, Jill Troup (Munns) '64-67, Beryl Warren (Allingham) '53-56, Norma Williams '58-61, Year of 1969-72.

Chapter 6

St. Andrew's Hospital	*Annual reports 1972 – 81*
St. Andrew's School of Occupational Therapy	*Archives 1972 – 81*
Student & Staff contributions	Lynne Gowen '72-75, Pat Harding '73-76 + current staff, Wendy Henry (staff '72-94), Helen O'Neill (Smith) '70-73, Carol Raffe (Atkinson) '70-73, Sara Simons '74-77 + current staff.

Chapter 7

Anon   *Northampton School and Nene College to merge* (BJOT, Oct 1992, 55, 10)
Cracknell, Elizabeth   *Personal papers 1981 – 95*
Indepen   *Report on market research project for the St. Andrew's Hospital School of Occupational Therapy* (1992)
NW Thames RHA   *Report on St. Andrew's Hospital School of Occupational Therapy* (1991)
St. Andrew's Hospital   *Annual reports 1981 – 95*
St. Andrew's School of Occupational Therapy   *Archives 1981 – 95*
Student and Staff contributions Lady Braye (committee chair 1986-2005), Elizabeth Cracknell (staff '81-95), Anna Fletcher '92-95, Pat Harding '73-76 + current staff, Sara Simons '74-77 + current staff, Year group '81-84

Chapters 8 & 9

Anon   *State of the art occupational therapy unit* (OT News, Oct 1997)
Kennard, S., N. Hayward & P.Paling   *The Princess Royal opens the School of Occupational Therapy, Nene* (St. Andrew's School of Occupational Therapy Friends Newsletter, 1998)
St. Andrew's School of Occupational Therapy   *Archives 1995 – 1998*
St. Andrew's School of Occupational Therapy Friends *Newsletters* (1999 – 2006)
Turner, Annie   *Moving on* (Insight, 1998)
Turner, Annie   *St. Andrew's School Farewell* (OT News, Feb 1998)
Student & Staff contributions   Lady Braye (committee chair 1986-2005), Dr. Susan Corr (current staff), Cheryl Corrodus '96-99, Sue Griffiths (current staff), Pat Harding '73-76 + current staff, Cormac Norton (current postgraduate), Cath Poyser (current postgraduate), Elleen Saunders (current student), Sara Simons '74-77 + current staff, Prof. Annie Turner (current staff), Beryl Warren '53-56, Sorrel Wilmer '98-02

Association of Occupational Therapists
Final examinations
1953
(5 questions to be attempted – 3 hours)

Psychiatry

1. What are the symptoms of general paralysis of the insane?
2. In what conditions do hypocondriacal symptoms occur? Give brief examples of each case.
3. What is delirium? Give some possible causes.
4. Cases have been referred to your Occupational therapy department who are
    a) Epileptics
    b) Having insulin treatment
    c) Having electric shock treatment

Describe the special precautions to be taken in each case.

5. Discuss the place of Hospital Utility Departments in the Occupational Therapy programme of a mental hospital.
6. Describe the personality changes following the operation of pre-frontal leucotomy, with special reference to behaviour in the Occupational Therapy Department.
7. Describe a case of obsessional neurosis.

Psychopathology

1. Discuss the psychopathology of the psychopathic deviation.
2. What is the part played by heredity in
    a) Mental Deficiency
    b) Manic-depressive Psychosis
    c) Schizophrenia
3. Discuss the psychopathology of drug addiction and alcoholism.
4. Explain what is meant by "Introspection" and give suitable examples.
5. Discuss the significance of hallucinations.
6. Differentiate between the terms "rapport" and "transference".
7. Describe the use of a projection test.

Occupational Therapy applied to Psychiatric Conditions

1. Discuss the relative value of individual and group Occupational Therapy with reference to different types of mental disorder.
2. What special problems would arise in carrying out Occupational Therapy with patients suffering from:-
    a) catatonic schizophrenia

      b) alcoholism
      c) hysteria
3. Outline your views on the organisation of a social club for neurotic patients, with special emphasis on the way in which it can aid recovery.
4. Why do you think it is important to consider a patient's mental capacity when planning occupational therapy? Illustrate your answer by examples from your own experience or observation.
5. Discuss the therapeutic value of any three of the following:-
      a) Play production   d) Modelling
      b) Weaving   e) Joinery
      c) Folk dancing   f) Gardening
6. Discuss whether you think a high standard of work should be insisted upon in Occupational Therapy, bearing in mind particularly the following:-
      a) a hypomanic patient
      b) a patient with obsessional neurosis
      c) a hysterical patient
      d) a patient with involutional depression.
7. Patients suffering from organic dementia tend to show a gradual deterioration of mental faculties and social instincts. Why is it important that such patients should be occupied and how would you set about organising occupational and recreational treatment for them?

Departmental Management

1. Design specimen case-cards for the treatment of patients in **one** of the following;
      TB Sanatorium, Mental Hospital, Rehabilitation Unit,
      Mental Deficiency Institution;
State briefly   a) whether you consider this to be important
                      b) from what sources you would expect to obtain your information.
2. You are required to order 12 pounds of rug wool for your department. Show how you would account for the use of this material from the time you placed the order to the sale of the finished articles.
3. You are asked to give treatment to 12 children in an orthopaedic ward. What crafts or other activities would you organise, and what tools and equipment would you consider essential for such a project?
4. Write brief notes giving your own views on **three** of the following:
      a) the use of drawing and painting in hospitals
      b) exhibitions and sales of work
      c) the employment of untrained personnel
      d) inter-departmental relations

5. You are asked to assist your hospital architect in the planning of your new department. State the points you would stress and give your reasons.
6. It is sometimes suggested that craft work might be supplemented by other activities in an Occupational Therapy Department. Give your views on this and list activities you consider suitable.
7. You are asked to plan the hospital practice for students in a general hospital. List the point you consider a) essential; b) desirable.

Applied Psychology

1. What special advantages are there for a patient a) in attempting something he has never done before, and b) in doing something which is familiar? Illustrate your answer by reference to cases where you would put the emphasis on these different aspects.
2. Discuss those aspects of the arrangement and equipment of an Occupational Therapy Department which you feel are most important from the point of view of their psychological effect upon the patients.
3. How would you differentiate between fatigue and boredom? Discuss probable signs and suitable treatment for each.
4. "It is never an individual who has to be treated but always a social group." Discuss this statement in the light of any observations you have made as to the influence of groups on individuals.
5. What special value do you think that Occupational Therapy may have for the very old? Discuss the special problems involved.
6. What different reasons may there be to account for the behaviour of a patient who is described as "solitary", "not a good mixer"? In order to help him, what principles would guide you a) in respecting his preference for being alone, and b) in encouraging him to be more sociable?
7. What in your experience are the chief incentives of which use may be made by an Occupational Therapist?

General Medicine and Surgery

1. A patient aged 30 years has disseminated sclerosis, describe the symptoms and signs she may have and discuss the treatment of the condition.
2. Discuss the causes of pain and swelling round the wrist joint.
3. A man aged 45 years complains of sudden pain in the chest whilst working in an Occupational Therapy Department, discuss the possible causes.
4. Write short notes on the following:-
    a) Heberdens Nodes
    b) Hallux Valgus

c) Tennis elbow
d) Coccydynia
5. An adult is coughing up blood stained sputum, what condition may cause this symptom and what investigations may be carried out in order to make a diagnosis.
6. How may acute rheumatism affect the heart during the attack and in later life? Give the pathological symptoms and signs.
7. Name two diseases caused by syphilis of the brain and spinal cord and describe one.

Anatomy and Physiology

1. Discuss how the body accommodates itself to a life at high altitudes.
2. Describe the left shoulder joint. Upon what does its stability depend?
3. What is the parasympathetic nervous system? What are its actions?
4. Describe how a long bone grows.
5. Describe the origin and course of the right sciatic nerve.
6. What is the pathway of a stretch reflex? (Knee jerk). Discuss the factors which influence it.
7. Describe the left scapula and its muscular attachments.

Occupational Therapy applied to Physical Conditions

1. Outline the ways in which the Occupational Therapy Department might assist in the resettlement of the disabled in the community.
2. A stevedore has a fractured mid-shaft of the right humerus, complicated by a radial nerve palsy. What part would Occupational Therapy play in his rehabilitation?
3. A housewife of 55 has had a right Radical Mastectomy for carcinoma of the breast. Describe a suitable course of Occupational Therapy.
4 A steam press operator sustained third degree burns of the left arm and hand which have now healed. There are contractures of the elbow, wrist and fingers. The patient is awaiting plastic surgery. What part will Occupational Therapy play before and after surgery.
5. Discuss the training of the paraplegic housewife in the activities of daily living and the running of her home. Indicate how you might co-operate with the physiotherapist and the almoner.
6. A window cleaner has a fractured os calcis. How will Occupational Therapy assist in his rehabilitation?
7. Discuss the role of Occupational Therapy in Paralysis Agitans (Parkinson's Disease).

Physical Medicine and Orthopaedics

1. Describe the Thomas Bed Knee Splint. Discuss in detail TWO conditions for which this splint may be used.
2. Describe in detail the symptoms and signs of osteoarthritis of the hip. Discuss the after treatment of a patient who has had an arthroplasty of the hip joint with particular reference to Occupational Therapy.
3. How does healing take place after fracture of a bone?
4. Write notes on:-
    a) Congenital dislocation of the hip.
    b) Fractures of the carpal scaphoid.
    c) Tennis elbow.
5. Mention THREE causes of low back ache. Discuss one of these conditions in detail.
6. What varieties of Motor Neurone Disease do you know? Describe one and suggest how the Occupational Therapist can help these patients.
7. Where are the common sites of injury to the ulnar nerve? Describe how an ulnar nerve lesion affects the function of the hand.

2006 Level 3 Assessment

Dissertation: 10,000 words based on an individual research project (primary or secondary research)
Professional Context: 1 seen exam paper (2 hours)
1 unseen exam paper (1 hour)
Professional Reasoning: Timed paper- 3,000 word assignment completed within a two week time period
Occupation for Health with Contributory Disciplines (OHCD):
Powerpoint Presentation (20 mins)
Viva (30 mins)
Practice – Profile: Assessment of competency during clinical practice placements

University of Northampton, School of Health, Division of Occupational Therapy

Spring 2006
Professional Context Exam
(Seen Paper)

You may take into the examination one piece of paper with type-written notes of up to 400 words detailing points, any quotations and the reference list on one side of A4. The notes will be checked before the exam and handed in with the answer. The answer should be properly referenced, observing normal Harvard referencing conventions. As the reference list is included in your type-written notes there is no need to re-write it in the exam. However, you may want to make amendments to reflect your answer.

Answer one question.
1 a) Explore the philosophy and policy leading to the proposed patient- led commissioning.
b) What impact could this have on an occupational therapy service?
2 The Sainsbury Centre for Mental Health (2004) recommends accurate data collection and the need for a whole systems approach on communication between in-patient and community teams. (OT News July 2005 p27)
a) Discuss what would be involved in a whole systems approach and how this could be introduced.

      b) Consider the implications for interprofessional working when a whole systems approach is introduced.
3   The NHS 'as the largest employer of black and minority ethnic staff, there is a moral duty to do things other organisations have not done.' (OT News July 2005 p26)
      a) Discuss ways in which the NHS is attempting to improve race equality.
      b) Select and evaluate an example of occupational therapy attempting to promote greater cultural understanding and integration.

Spring 2006
Professional Context Exam
(Unseen Paper) 1 hour

You must answer all of this question.

You are a newly qualified band 5 occupational therapist and you are working in a busy large hospital. You have concerns that a fellow newly qualified OT is not completing their documentation, and have witnessed them taking notes home with them.

Outline the ethical issues that this poses, what are the wider implications and how do you act.

(This paper is designed to test the student's intuitive reactions to ethical issues and their ability to articulate clinical judgements.)

Some Eminent Alumni and Staff of the Northampton School of Occupational Therapy

We have defined 'eminent' as former students who have been made Fellows of the College of Occupational Therapy, who have been asked to give the Casson Memorial Lecture, who have been elected Chairman of Council at C.O.T., or who have become a Head of School.

Fellows are occupational therapists who have made an outstanding contribution to the development of OT practice and given special service to the profession, for example, in research, practice or teaching. Casson Memorial Lecturers are selected for the way in which their thinking has contributed to occupational therapy. Chairmen of Council are members of the profession who show great vision and leadership skills.

Dr. Rosemary E. Barnitt BSc, MSc, PhD, DipCOT, SROT

Rosemary Barnitt graduated from St. Andrew's School of Occupational Therapy in 1964 and began her career at the Children's Hospital in Adelaide, South Australia. Returning to the UK she worked in research before studying for a BSc in Psychology and an MSc in Occupational Psychology. In 1981 Rosemary was appointed Principal of the Liverpool College of Occupational Therapy and then in 1992 led the new School of Occupational Therapy and Physiotherapy at the University of Southampton, where she was awarded a personal chair in 2001. Over the years, Rosemary has delivered a number of keynote speeches, including the 1991 Casson Memorial Lecture, *Through a Glass, Darkly,* reflecting her interest in education.. Regarded as one of the pioneers in the field of research, she is an active member of the multi-professional Society for Research and Rehabilitation. In 1996 she was awarded a PhD for her thesis, *An investigation of ethical dilemmas in Occupational Therapy and Physiotherapy: Issues of methodology and practice.* She was proud to be awarded a Fellowship of the C.O.T. in 1998. Rosemary retired in 2003 but continues to do research and in 2004 was supervising four doctoral students.

Kay East DipCOT (née Smith)

Kay qualified at St. Andrew's School of Occupational Therapy in 1967 and has worked as a clinician and manager in health and social services. She has been involved in policy development in a local authority, in education as a university lecturer, and in the voluntary sector as a member of her local Community Health Council. At a national level, Kay has been a member of the Government's Modernisation Action Team and in 2002 was a member of the Older People's Task Force. She was elected Chairman of the C.O.T. Council in 1999. In 2002 Kay was appointed as Chief Health Professions Officer at the Department of Health – a new role which recognised the contribution of AHPs and was designed to raise their profile. Kay retired in 2006.

E. Naomi Fraser-Holland BA, PhD, TdipCOT, AFBPsS, RGN, CPA, FRSH (née Dunkin)
Dr. Naomi Fraser-Holland began training at the St. Andrew's School of Occupational Therapy in 1950. She has also trained as a nurse, physiotherapist and psychologist, as well as holding a C.O.T. training diploma. In 1953 she began her occupational therapy career in Canada, following a period of teaching at McGill University, where there was a joint physiotherapy and occupational therapy course. In 1962 she came to join the St. Loyes School of Occupational Therapy, Exeter, as a senior tutor, and was awarded her PhD in Psychology (Human Learning) in 1971. She continued as senior tutor at St. Loyes until 1985, when she became a research fellow and coordinator of the multidisciplinary MSc at the University of Exeter. Throughout the 1980s and 1990s she served on many C.O.T. committees. In 1990 she gave the Casson Memorial Lecture, entitled *Moving Targets and 20:20 Vision*, which was concerned with the history of training for the profession. In 1998 she was appointed to the post of Course Director / Senior Lecturer at London Hospital Medical College and London University School of Occupational Therapy.

Ruth Heames MA, DipCOT, SROT, Dip Ed, Cert Ed   (née Boocock)
Ruth qualified at St. Andrew's in 1976, and after working in various posts returned to the School as a student teacher, becoming a lecturer in 1983. Having been appointed Senior Lecturer at Coventry Polytechnic (now Coventry University), she became Head of the Occupational Therapy Department in 1995. Her particular research interests lie in curriculum design and development, profiling, and teaching and learning methods. Ruth's professional activities include time as an external examiner and work on the Joint Validation Committee of the C.O.T. Her latest publication is 'Managing the Pressures in Teaching: Practical Ideas for Tutors and their Students' (1999). She has subsequently made numerous presentations to conferences.

Joan E. Martin TDipCOT, MA, DPhil
Joan Martin graduated from the St. Andrew's School in 1972. She first worked at King's College Hospital and then at Atkinson Morley Hospital. There she became interested in anorexia nervosa and did a considerable amount of work to develop treatment programmes. In 1979 she qualified as a teacher, gaining both the CNAA Certificate in Education and the C.O.T. teaching diploma. In 1981 she was awarded a Fellowship by Examination of the C.O.T. for her thesis entitled *The art of treating*

Anorexia Nervosa: the condition, the different treatment models and the role of occupational therapy. She returned home to Northern Ireland and began her teaching career at the University of Ulster. In 1986 she was awarded an MA from Warwick University for her thesis, *Bulimia Nervosa: an exploration of its social origins.* She continued her scholastic journey gaining a DPhil through published works from the University of Ulster, and is thought to be the first occupational therapist in the UK to do so.

Dr. Maralynne D. Mitcham

is currently Professor and Director of the Occupational Therapy Programme at the Department of Rehabilitation Sciences, College of Health Professions, Medical University of South Carolina. She gained her Diploma from St. Andrew's School, her Bachelor of Science and Master of Health Education degrees from the Medical College of Georgia, and her PhD in educational psychology from the University of Georgia. In the clinical arena, Dr. Mitcham has worked in adult rehabilitation, prevocational evaluation, and gerontology. She is a recent past president of the American Occupational Therapy Foundation. Recipient of many honours and awards, in 2006 she received a Recognition of Achievement award from the American Occupational Therapy Association for advancing occupational therapy education through faculty development.

Professor Ann Turner DipCOT, MA, FCOT

After qualifying as an occupational therapist, Ann Turner worked in Oswestry, Leicester and Derby, before spending a couple of years in the British Voluntary Programme in Honduras. She was Head Occupational Therapist at Battle Hospital, Reading between 1973 and 1975 before moving into the area of education. She worked first at St. Loyes, Exeter, and then at St. Andrew's School where she became Divisional Leader of Occupational Therapy in 1996 when the School became part of University College Northampton. Ann made a major contribution to the profession through her editorship of *Occupational Therapy and Physical Dysfunction: Principles, Skills and Practice (Edinburgh: Harcourt Publications, 2002),* which is now in its fifth edition. She was influential at a national level as a member of C.O.T. Council and as a member of its Education and Practice Board. In 2000 she was awarded a Fellowship of the C.O.T. In 2006 she took on a new role at the University, becoming the professional lead in the Division. Part of this work has involved developing an Open University foundation course for occupational therapy. In 2007 the University of Northampton awarded her the title of Professor of Occupational Therapy in recognition of the contribution she has made to the profession.

Beryl Warren DipCOT (née Allingham)
Beryl qualified at St. Andrew's School of Occupational Therapy in 1956 and worked for several years in a hospital for neurological diseases and then in psychiatry. In 1976 she became the Head O.T. at the Wolfson Medical Rehabilitation Centre and District O.T. for Wandsworth Health Authority. She was seconded to the DHSS as assistant O.T. Officer for a year and moved to a Social Services Department as Principal Officer for Physical and Sensory Disability, later becoming Service Manager for older people and people with disabilities. She retired from practice in 1993.For many years Beryl took an active part in the running of the profession, eventually becoming a nationally elected member of B.A.O.T. and Vice Chairman of Council. She was an alternate member of the Occupational Therapy Board of the C.P.S.M. and a member of the C.O.T. Professional & Ethical Committee, becoming its chairman in 1986 and again in 1991. In 1986 she was elected Chairman of B.A.O.T./C.O.T. Council at a difficult time when the profession was facing industrial disputes at its headquarters. Since retirement her main activity has been the foundation and development of the Friends of St Andrew's School of Occupational Therapy (the Friends of Occupational Therapy Education Northampton) after the School moved to Park Campus at the University of Northampton in 1997.